THE TALE OF A FIST-SIZED HOLE

TRAVIS MCGINNIS

The Tale of a Fist-Sized Hole

Travis McGinnis

Cover Art By:
Brandon Philbrick

Edited By:
Mavis Ness
Becky Guimont

ISBN-13: 978-1517732349
ISBN-10: 1517732344

For Grandpa Bernard.
He passed away from skin cancer in 1958.

For Uncle Bruce.
He passed away from pancreatic cancer in 1998.

For Uncle Greg.
He passed away from prostate cancer in 2015.

For my wife, Kayleigh.
You are my rock. My voice of reason.
I never would have made it through this without you.
I love you more than life itself.

Acknowledgments

Special thanks to Dr. Thomas Wyne, Dr. Daniel Lachance, Dr. Fred Meyer, Dr. Scott Stafford, Dr. Donald Jurgens, and Nealy Cray, CNP.

Also thanks to every other doctor, nurse, and medical professional who has cared for me during this journey.

Finally, thank you to The Hope Lodge in Rochester.

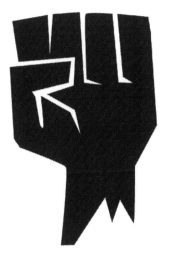

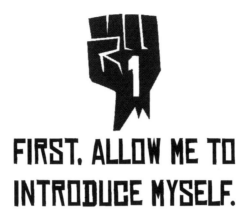

FIRST, ALLOW ME TO INTRODUCE MYSELF.

I wrote this book to not only share my story about brain cancer, but also to inspire people and make you laugh a little bit along the way. I believe joy can be found in all things, even cancer. I also find it helps me cope when I write down my thoughts. This book is a collection of my journal entries, blog posts, and Caring Bridge updates over the last year or so. I've edited them together and added some other tidbits along the way.

This book is for anyone who has battled cancer or has a family member who has fought cancer. Whether they've won or lost their fight is irrelevant. My hope is that within these pages you'll find hope and laughter. It is also for anyone looking for a good pick-me-up. I know, it sounds weird to use that phrase in a cancer book, but I promise you it's in here.

Fair warning. I'm going to get a little graphic in parts of this book. I don't mean to gross you out, but those little details are important to understand what I was going through at the time. If you're grossed out by vomit, diarrhea, blood, and other natural bodily functions, you've been warned. So don't get mad at me for not giving a disclaimer.

So, let's get started.

My name is Travis Bernard McGinnis. I was born at a very young age in November of 1983. I'm the son of a toilet salesman and a secretary. I'm kidding. My parents work in plumbing and heating wholesale. So yes, they really do sell toilets, among many other things. Mom is a purchasing agent, though she started her career as a secretary. Dad does commercial plumbing quotations. When I was a kid, he was an on-the-road salesman for many years.

They met on the job, dated, and got married. Definitely not your typical workplace romance by any stretch of the imagination. Most workplace romances end shortly after they begin and result in office awkwardness with fake smiles, while trying to avoid each other in the breakroom. Lucky for me, it worked out for them. I owe my life to it. Literally.

My parents and my wife's parents are still married to this day. We both have great examples of what a happy, healthy, and successful marriage looks like.

My middle name is after my grandpa Barney. He was a full-blooded Irishman. He passed away from melanoma in 1958 – my dad wasn't even two years old. Yet, from what Dad tells me, he was a great man, a loving husband, and a devoted father. I bet he would have been an amazing grandpa too.

So yes, I'm Irish and damn proud of it! Though it does get annoying when I tell someone my last name and they ask, "McGinnis...like the beer?"

"Yes, like the beer," I reply, "but spelled differently." It happens all the time. Good thing I like Guinness.

I have two younger siblings: a brother and a sister named Aaron and Michaela. Growing up, my life was pretty good. I didn't get into any serious trouble; I didn't drink or smoke or stay out past eleven.

Okay, I lied. I smoked once. I took two puffs on a cigarette and started coughing uncontrollably. The person who gave it to me exclaimed, "Don't worry! The next one is better!" *Better!?* I thought. I don't know why anyone would ever go for a "next one" if the first one was so awful. But I digress. I'm getting off track.

I married at the young age of 22 to a gorgeously awesome gal named Kayleigh. We have three beautiful daughters together. At the time of this writing, they are Alexis (11), Tatum (5), and Harper (1). If you're doing the math, yes, we had sex before we got married. Shame on us. That's probably the most risqué thing I've done in my life; I'm such a rebel.

I also have two female cats. So yes, I'm surrounded by women, but I wouldn't have it any other way. I love my girls more than life itself. (With the exception of the cats. I love my life more than I love the cats.) In fact, we ever have a son, I'm not sure I would know what to do with him. I've got this whole raising girls thing figured out. At least 5% of it for sure. Granted, they're not at the whole teenage-boy-crazy-periods-tampons-run-to-the-store-for-pads-emotional-mood-swing stage yet.

I work for a small, local company called Leighton Interactive. It's the Inbound Marketing Agency division of Leighton Enterprises, which also owns several radio stations under the name Leighton Broadcasting. That's where I got my start in 2005. I was a part time on-air host for Wild Country 99, and full-time Production Director when off-air.

My on-air moniker was JT. "Why JT?" you ask. Well, there's a longer story here than I'd care to admit. The program director for the station asked what I wanted my on-air name to be.

"What's wrong with just Travis?" I asked.

He thought about it for a second. A smile crept across his face. Then, out of nowhere, he exclaimed, "I've got it! We'll call you JT! Just Travis! Get it!" Then proceeded to laugh hysterically at his own stupid joke.

When you say it, though, you need to really get into it. Bend your knees, spread your legs shoulder distance apart and wave your hands with excitement. Use your spirit fingers. Try it with me.

Just Travis!

Not so much? I guess you'd have to see it in person. It's just one of those things that are better in person.

The name stuck. I was on-air as "JT" for several years. Even after I stopped being on-air, the nickname followed me. I haven't been on the radio since 2008, but still to this day, folks call me JT. I guess I must look like a JT.

In 2009, we started Leighton Interactive. It was just one of our sales guys, Dan, and me. In April of the following year, we hired a guy named Brandon to be our graphic designer, thus rounding out our needs for a sales guy,

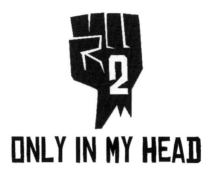

ONLY IN MY HEAD

I had my first episode - or as I would later find out, my first seizure - in February of 2014.

My wife asked me something as I walked downstairs. That's when it happened. I was digging for something in the basement closet. I had this tingly sensation across the front of my forehead, kind of like when your foot falls asleep, but only in my head. Not on the surface either. I felt it *inside* my head. I've never experienced anything like it before. It didn't hurt at all; it just felt weird to have a sensation like that in my head.

I also had these really bizarre thoughts about what she told me and what was going on around me. It's hard to explain what those thoughts were, because I cannot replicate them after the episode is done. My doctors would later call it an "unusual phychosensory experience."

From what I can remember, I felt like I had discovered an awesome new super power. The power to make people say whatever I wanted them to say, but only in my head. It was like I could control them, but only in my head. I could make them say curse words, but only in my head. This

particular instance, I had imagined my wife saying "shit."
My wife *never* swears, so I thought it was awesome that I
could make her say *shit* if I wanted to. But only in my
head. During each seizure, I felt awesome because I could
control what people would say to me ... but only in my
head.

In every episode, I followed the same thought process:
take what someone is saying to me at the moment and
make them say something else. I thought I had a super
power.

If it wasn't that, I would have really bizarre thoughts
about what they were saying to me and how I interpreted
their words. These are the thoughts I cannot replicate; they
were gone as soon as the seizure was over.

Obviously, anyone can think what they want about
someone else and there's nothing that person can do about
it. For some reason though, while I was having a seizure, it
felt like I had some nifty new super power.

It sounds silly when I read those words back to myself,
because it's not a super power at all. Stupid is what it is.
During a seizure though, I felt like I could control the words
of people. It was awesome and stupid at the same time.

The second seizure was with my soon-to-be middle
daughter, Tatum. My wife was pregnant during all of this,
due to have our third daughter in early May. It was a breezy
March day. Tatum and I were walking into the house when
the seizure hit.

I remember getting very angry at her for no reason at all.
I didn't say anything because I knew she hadn't done
anything wrong. She didn't deserve to get scolded for
something she didn't do. And yet, I was angry.

Again, I made her swear in my head. (I'm not sure why most of my episodes had to do with making people swear in my head.) I set her down and took my shoes off. I kept quiet, kept to myself.

Each episode only lasted for 10-15 seconds, but they felt much longer.

The third episode was in early April. I had just gotten back from DJ'ing a show out of town. I had a side gig as a DJ for weddings, teen dances, corporate parties, etc. It was well past midnight. As my trainee and I were unloading the equipment at the warehouse in downtown St. Cloud, another co-worker, Darren, was already there unloading his gear.

Darren and I made small talk about our shows and the way he had his setup. He was doing a bigger show for a teen dance, so he had to bring two amplifiers and daisy chain some speakers together. This let the sound make it all around the gymnasium. He explained that the guy who was in charge of the dance was really annoying. A techie "know-it-all" kind of guy. This guy wanted to hook up his gear to Darren's gear to get the sound bigger and louder.

I asked how many people were at his show. "Probably 500 or so," he answered. That's when the seizure started. He then asked how many people were at my show.

When I tried to reply, my speech wouldn't work. I knew what I wanted to say: *About 300 people.* Instead, I just stuttered.

"Ah-eh-ih-eh-ah." Those were the only sounds I could muster. It was terrifying. Both Darren and my trainee heard me stutter. They didn't know what to say, because everything *looked* normal, but I was having a seizure. It was a difficult few seconds afterwards, but it felt like an eternity of embarrassment.

Eventually, Darren awkwardly spoke, "Well, okay then. Have a good night."

I responded as if nothing had happened. I was embarrassed. They saw the one thing I was trying to hide, to keep a secret. Secretly hoping would never happen again. They saw the whole thing. I was terrified. I had no idea what was wrong with me.

I knew something wasn't right. I figured the first two episodes were just random things that happen as you get older. When my speech was interrupted, I knew something major was wrong.

I thought about it the entire drive home. I was scared out of my mind. I didn't think much about what it might mean. In fact, the words "tumor" and "cancer" never once crossed my mind. It was close to 1:00 a.m. when I got home. Kayleigh was long asleep. I was tempted to wake her and tell her what had just happened, but I opted to wait until morning.

I didn't sleep very well that night. When the sun finally broke the darkness, I knew it was morning. I laid there until Kayleigh's alarm went off.

I told her before we even got out of bed.

"Something happened last night when I was dropping the gear off." I continued to tell her the whole story.

"You should talk to your doctor," she advised.

Luckily, my annual physical was less than a month away.

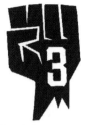

THE MRI THAT SAVED MY LIFE

"You can never be too cautious when it comes to the brain," explained Dr. Wyne, "I think we should get an MRI done. You know, just in case." His name is pronounced *wine*, like the alcoholic beverage.

I had just finished telling him about the three episodes I had experienced in the previous months. I focused mainly on the third one when my speech was interrupted, as that was the most frightening.

Dr. Wyne has been my family doctor for as long as I can remember. My parents took us kids to see him before we were even old enough to walk. He spoke softly, and had a genuine smile behind his thin white beard. He looked like a skinny Santa Claus with a doctor's coat and a stethoscope around his neck. Every year, he gave me the same piece of advice: Cherish your wife. Take her on dates. Respect your parents. Listen to their advice.

"It's probably just stress," he went on, "Have you been experiencing any stress lately?"

I laughed to myself. My wife and I had been going through quite the ordeal with her pregnancy. We found out just a couple of months prior to this about a condition she had called Placenta Previa, but the doctors also suspected a condition known as Vasa Previa. They did a Level 3 Ultrasound to verify if that was the case. Thankfully, it was not. She just had Placenta Previa.

This is a complication where her placenta entirely covers (major) or partially covers (minor) the birth canal. Hers was classified as major because it nearly covered the entire opening to the birth canal.

She had ultrasounds every few weeks to see if the Previa was still present. It'll often correct itself by the third trimester. Hers, unfortunately, didn't correct itself, so we had to keep checking every couple of weeks.

The chances of it going away during the third-trimester were pretty much non-existent. If she went into labor naturally, the baby's life would be in serious danger. It was almost guaranteed that she'd need to have the baby via cesarean section, and it would have to happen a couple weeks before the due date to ensure she didn't start labor naturally.

We checked one last time at the appointment where we were going to schedule the date of the C-section. Miraculously, it was gone. Kayleigh's doctor was dumbfounded. Never in her career had she seen something like that. Kayleigh was just over 36 weeks along and they couldn't find anything.

On May 12th, 2014, we welcomed Harper Rowan McGinnis into the world via a natural birth.

After I explained what we were going through, Dr. Wyne just smiled and nodded. "Yep, I'd call that stressful!" he half joked.

"You know, many of my colleagues wouldn't order this MRI," he continued.

"Why not?" I asked.

"Because you don't have any other symptoms we typically look for to signify something might be wrong with the brain."

"What type of symptoms?" I enquired, wondering to myself if I had any of them, but not really thinking anything of it.

"Well, there's headaches, nausea and/or vomiting, ringing in the ears, blurry vision. Those are some of the main ones; they're physical signs that something might be wrong with the brain."

I was relieved.

"I haven't had any of those," I quickly replied.

"Which is why it's probably stress. But let's get an MRI done just to be safe."

Dr. Wyne saved my life when he ordered that MRI.

The MRI took forever to get scheduled. I actually had to call the clinic three times before they got me on their calendar. I had my physical on May 5th, 2014. The MRI didn't happen until June 27th, nearly two months later. Apparently, from what I was told, the nurse never put in the doctor's order for an MRI. When she finally did, the MRI place missed it, hence the multiple phone calls to get it booked.

Plus, I kept putting off calling because I would go a few weeks without an episode. I'd think that I was all better. Then I'd have a seizure, and I'd call to ask about the MRI.

I continued to have episodes until my MRI on June 27th. It was about one episode per month or so.

We had an event at work where I had the pleasure to speak in front of a group of clients, potential clients, and industry peers. It was our first ever 100 Proof Happy Hour. As an Inbound Marketing Agency with a progressive culture, we can have fun with our event names. We served appetizers and my very own homebrewed beer. We talked about inbound marketing and how it can bring results for a business.

I was terrified I would have an episode in front of them. I didn't want to lose my train of thought and not be able to speak. At that point nobody at work knew what was going on. I wasn't going to tell anyone until I had something to tell. I was nervous the entire time leading up to my turn to speak. Time moved in slow motion as the seconds slowly ticked away into minutes.

"And now, our Director of Marketing Services, Travis McGinnis," my boss introduced me.

The group applauded as I took my place at the front of the room and began my presentation about how Inbound Marketing is a lot like brewing your own beer. Every business has their own unique recipe required to deliver results. Our Creative Director designed an impressive infographic to visually show this analogy.

As I began speaking, I got more and more comfortable. I fell into a rhythm. I didn't even notice the clock on the wall as the time ticked by.

Then, it happened.

I was done. My part of the presentation was over. No seizures, only a round of applause from the audience. The event went off without a hitch. It was a big success and seizure free for me. Plus, my homebrew was quite the hit!

I don't remember the order of the episodes that happened after my physical in May, but I recall each one rather vividly.

I had one episode where my boss called me on the phone to ask about some content on one of our websites. I had an episode just as he called. I couldn't think of what to say because of the seizure. So I just told him to hold on while I "take a look."

I blamed the internet for being slow, but I was just buying time until the episode passed. He didn't seem to notice anything. I couldn't think straight during that particular episode. I had no idea what to say, though I was, at least, capable of speaking. I had to wait until the seizure was done before I could answer his questions.

Another episode I had at work was when a client called. She had questions about a Facebook promotion they wanted to run again. That time my speech was affected as well. I was only able to mutter "Umm....ummm...umm," until the episode passed. Afterwards, I made an excuse that I was reading something else and I apologized for not paying more attention to her question. That seemed to go over smoothly, because she didn't act awkward at all. We continued the conversation as if nothing had happened.

Some episodes were very minor, some were fairly major. But none like the one I had at the warehouse late that night where my speech was interrupted. I recall one minor episode, again at work, where we had just wrapped up a meeting in the conference room. Everyone else was leaving, but I sat there for a few seconds until it passed. I then got up and walked quietly back to my office. I sat at my desk for a few minutes, thinking about what just happened. Nobody ever seemed to notice, so I don't know if I had a look on my face while I was having a seizure. I imagine my eyes glazed over and it looked like I was staring off into the distance.

Then I called the clinic again to inquire about the MRI they missed twice already. I finally had an appointment on the books.

Once we had the MRI scheduled, we decided to tell our parents. It would have sucked for the scan to find something and then have to tell them not only about the MRI, but the episodes I was experiencing that led up to it, *plus* the fact that it found something. That's a lot of bad news to take in one sitting.

We asked them not to tell anyone else until we knew more.

June 27th, 2014

I went to the MRI on a Friday afternoon with my wife and newborn daughter, Harper. It was on the main floor of the St. Cloud Hospital. The halls were eerily quiet, a ghost town. We made small talk as we meandered through the corridors to the imaging lab.

There was a lone clerk at the desk where I checked in. We were the only ones down there, so the wait wasn't long. The MRI tech called me back after a few minutes. I gave Kayleigh a kiss and shot her the "wish me luck" look. Then I walked towards the MRI room. I've never had an MRI before. My heart rate was increasing. I was shaking and cold. My hands were clammy.

The tech led me to a changing room. He instructed me to strip down to my underwear, put on a hospital gown, and make sure I had no metal on me at all.

"What about my wedding ring?" I asked.

He chuckled as if he gets that question all the time. "That'll be fine. You might feel it vibrate, but that's about it."

I took it off anyways, just to be safe.

If you've never seen an MRI machine, imagine a giant white tube about 6 feet in diameter and 10 feet long. Long enough to fit an entire person for full-body MRI scans. In the middle, there's a hole just barely large enough for a fully grown adult.

I laid on the table as the tech put earplugs in and secured my head. He asked if I would like a blanket. I declined, which I later regretted since it was ice-cold in the MRI room.

The table was raised up and it slid me head first into the tube. Good thing I'm not claustrophobic; it was a tight fit. I kept my fingers clenched around the emergency stop button he gave me. I looked around the best I could since my head was restrained. The inside of the machine was all white. There were scuff marks in a few places. Just above my head, there was a white circle. It blended in with the rest of the interior, but stood out enough that I could see it. I figured this is what I was being lined up with.

I heard some loud clicking noises as the machine spun up. I can't even begin to describe the noises those machines make. Since I was inside, I could hear and feel the magnets moving around my white tomb. High pitched. Low pitched. Vibrating laser sounds. The noise was nearly constant, with only small moments of peace between each scan. The scans had a unique noise pattern that would repeat over and over. Some scans lasted only a few seconds, while others were several minutes long.

I'd find myself moving my eyes or blinking to the pattern of the noises. I'd wiggle a toe with the pattern, or tap my fingers. Anything to make the time go by faster and to keep my mind occupied since the white landscape in front of me was so bland and boring.

About half-way through, the tech stopped the machine and gave me an injection of a chemical called gadolinium contrast medium. Or just "contrast" for short. He injected it in the vein in the crook of my elbow. I could actually *hear* it entering my arm and the back of my neck as the drug moved through my spine. "Awkward" is the best word to describe the sensation of contrast moving through my body. Contrast makes certain tissues or abnormalities more visible on the MRI pictures. It also makes high grade tumors show up more brightly.

All in all, the scan took about 45 minutes. I was so cold,

I was shivering uncontrollably as the procedure finished. I was anxious to get my clothes back on and to see my wife.

We were waiting in the lobby for a while afterwards. Looking back, I realize they made us wait because they found something. If they hadn't, they would have sent us on our merry way to call later with the results.

I got the results over the phone. "The MRI shows a mass about three centimeters by six centimeters in the front left of your brain," the doctor explained. I was stoic. I don't remember the rest of the conversation, but there wasn't much else to it. They wanted me to come in at a later date for a biopsy to figure out what it was and what to do with it if it turned out to be anything serious.

In a heartbeat, my life was flipped-turned upside down; and not in the "moving with your auntie and uncle in Bel Air" kind of way, either. That's not the kind of news you get every day, and there's no possible way to prepare for it.

What could it be? I wondered. *They didn't say tumor, or cancer. They just called it a mass. That's got to be good, right?*

When I hung up the phone, I turned and walked toward my wife. Time moved in slow motion. She was still in the waiting area about 15 feet away with our baby in the stroller.

I sat down next to her. Motionless. In shock.

"They found a mass." I told her.

"You're kidding, right?" she replied quickly.

"I wouldn't joke about something like that."

We both sat in silence for a few moments before getting up and walking towards the car. We talked about what it could possibly be. We decided not to worry until we knew for sure. Much easier said than done.

On the way out, I called my parents to tell them. They answered right away - almost as if they were expecting me to call. Can you blame them? I'd be nervous too if I were them.

I could tell my mom was starting to choke up, so she passed the phone off to Dad. They said they'd pray for us and to keep them updated. Then we headed back to Kayleigh's parents' house. Most of the drive was spent in contemplative silence. It hadn't quite sunk in yet.

There was a big annual parade that night, part of the Sauk Rapids River Days. Since Kayleigh's parents live on the parade route, they host a get-together every year for friends and family. Everyone brings a dish to share; we fire up the grill and have a cookout. There's a huge spread of food and drinks. Every year, we end up with leftovers. It's something we've done for a long time, even as far back to when Kayleigh and I were dating. It became one of our annual family traditions.

I walked in through the back door and sat on the couch. Kayleigh walked around the side of the house to the front. She made eye contact with her mom and started tearing up. They both came inside and Kayleigh shared the news with her parents and youngest sister, Sophia.

Eventually, we made it back outside to watch the parade and have some time with our kids. It was a good distraction for a little while.

That night, I made phone calls to my close friends and family to share the news. It was their shaky voices and choked reactions that made reality set in. I collapsed on my bedroom floor weeping.

My thoughts were a rollercoaster of morbidity and positivity.

"I don't want you to be alone," I cried to my wife as she wept too.

"Nobody is thinking that, Honey," she replied. "We'll get through this."

You know what? She's right. I know she is. This will be something I can look back on years from now as a terrible speed bump in an otherwise amazing and joyful life.

It took us a while to compose ourselves. At least the kids were sleeping. We just laid on the floor in each other's arms. Eventually, we decided move to the bed so we could try to sleep.

We had a big day in the morning.

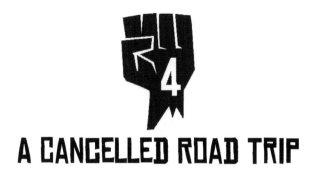

A CANCELLED ROAD TRIP

The MRI was on a Friday evening. On Saturday, we went to the annual Sauk Rapids River Days Food Fest at a local park. There were thousands of people, and tons of great food. None of it good for you, but where's the fun in that? The event had live music on stage, a beer garden, and bouncy-houses for kids. That was the other event we made a point to attend every year.

That evening, we drove up to Fargo to visit some friends for their daughter's baptism the next day.

After the baptism on Sunday morning, we headed further north to Grand Forks, North Dakota. Kayleigh's home town. She had family up there who we rarely get to see. We were going to spend a couple of days up there visiting her family. We both took Monday and Tuesday off from work.

When we arrived on Sunday evening, we had dinner, did some swimming at the hotel, and went to bed. We decided not to tell kids about the MRI findings until we knew more.

The next morning, Monday, I got a call from the hospital. Their on-call neurologist looked at my MRI scan and wanted me to head home right away. Based on the location of the tumor, I could seizure at any moment.

That's when we told the girls.

We sat them down on the bed and spoke quietly.

"Daddy has a bump in his head," we explained softly, trying to make it easy for Tatum to understand. She had just turned four a few days prior to.

Alexis, on the other hand, asked right away, "Does Daddy have cancer?" Her eyes welled up with tears. She started weeping uncontrollably. Not knowing what was going on, and sensing that something really bad was happening, Tatum started crying, too.

"We don't know, Honey," Kayleigh told her. "That's why we need to go back to St. Cloud. They're going to put Daddy on some medicine that will help. They also need to cut a piece of it out to find out what it is."

I figured I should probably tell my boss. He didn't answer the first few times, so I sent him a text:

Call me please. It's urgent.

He called within minutes. I told him about the MRI and what they found.

Stunned silence. He was at a loss for words. His life had just changed too. One of his management team members, and a friend at that, had a brain tumor. Our company wasn't big enough to handle that kind of situation. We didn't have the staff to fill in for my duties.

I told him it was okay to tell everyone at the office. It

wasn't a secret anymore. He said he'd start with the CEO, and the rest of the leadership team.

All of this happened while the kids were getting their swimsuits on to head down to the hotel pool. We had to pack up right away, cancel our trip and head back home. It was a 3 ½ hour drive back to St. Cloud. With two more nights left on the hotel reservation, I was prepared to pay for both nights.

I didn't.

I think the hotel concierge could sense something major was wrong with the tone of my voice when I told her I had an emergency and needed to cancel our next two nights. She said that wouldn't be a problem.

We packed our things as fast as humanly possible, and headed back to St. Cloud. I was told not to drive in case I had a seizure while on the road. Kayleigh took the wheel on the way back home.

I received text messages from most of my co-workers in the minutes and hours that followed. Each message had words of encouragement; telling me that we were in their thoughts and prayers.

I spent the trip texting and calling friends I didn't speak to the night we found out. I wanted to let them know what was going on.

When we arrived in St. Cloud a few hours later, we dropped the kids off at Kayleigh's parents, and headed to the emergency room.

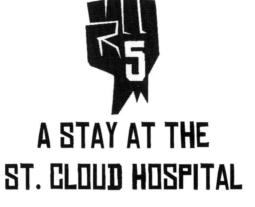

A STAY AT THE
ST. CLOUD HOSPITAL

They checked me in for two days. They wanted to run some tests.

First they did an electroencephalogram – don't try to pronounce it. I tried. It's impossible. That's why it's called an EEG for short. It was actually kind of trippy. The tech connected all sorts of sensors to my head with sticky goop. That took a good 20 minutes to get me wired up. Then she shut the lights off and put a strobe light in front of my face.

"Don't open your eyes," I was instructed.

The strobe made all sorts of funky patterns that I could see through my eyelids. I felt like I was on acid. Not that I've ever done acid. But like I said, it was trippy. The test took about a half hour. It came back normal.

Then, they ran advanced blood tests to make sure there wasn't an infection anywhere that would show up in my blood work.

Then came the spinal tap. No, not the awesomely awful 80's biopic.

I've heard horror stories about spinal taps. I was scared out of my mind. I pictured a super thick, 12-inch long needle stabbing into my spinal cord to extract spinal fluid. Even though pain killers are used, they don't affect the spine itself. The doctors can't actually see where they're trying to go, so they just dig around with the needle until it hits a pocket between vertebrae where the liquid gold they seek is hiding.

It was nothing like that at all.

The needle was (only) 6 inches long, and not nearly as thick as I had imagined. They numbed up the area, too. All of this happened on an X-ray table. Once my spine was lined up, they placed a pair of metal scissors on my back so it would show up on the X-ray picture. They positioned the pointy end on the spot to insert the needle. They marked it with a pen, then removed the scissors. The whole X-ray thing was a brilliant way to do a spinal tap. It was over in a matter of minutes. No pain at all. So much for those damn horror stories I'd heard.

All of these tests were to rule out any other possibilities, like a viral infection. They all came back normal.

While in the hospital, I spoke to a neurosurgeon. I learned that when it comes to brain tumors, they don't take any chances. A full surgical extraction is always what they do first. No wasting time on a biopsy. That will happen after the tumor comes out.

"I can certainly take it out here," he explained. "But if you were my kid, I'd rather have the best possible treatment, especially at your age."

I was referred down to the Mayo Clinic in Rochester, which was, thankfully, fully covered by my insurance.

It's Not Official until it's Facebook Official

Once the visit date for the Mayo was set, my wife and I decided to make the news "Facebook Official." I made this post while in the hospital on July 1st:

So since I post good news on Facebook, I might as well post the bad.

I had an MRI last Friday and they found a tumor on the left side of my brain. It's about 3cm x 6cm.

I was admitted to the hospital yesterday on seizure watch and to get more tests done.

My neurologist has referred me to the Mayo Clinic to likely get surgery to remove the tumor and hopefully return to life as normal.

The neurologist classified it as a "low grade malignant tumor." So yes, technically its cancer, but in the sense that any abnormal growth of cells is considered cancerous. My neurologist has no reason to believe that it is aggressive or that it is fast growing...no signs so far point to that.

I had a spinal tap today to eliminate other possibilities like a bacterial infection.

My Mayo appointment is next Thursday the 10th.

Aside from the fact that I have a brain tumor, I feel 100% normal. No pain, no discomfort. Life is great.

Thoughts and prayers are appreciated more than you'll ever know.

The post had 15 likes, 6 shares and 72 comments within a few days of going up. I had a lot of support.

In the handful of posts we made about the issue in the first few weeks, the outpouring of comments, likes, shares and positivity has moved us to tears many times.

I've had family members offer up their homes during our traveling back and forth to the Mayo.

A friend from high school messaged me and shared her story about her battle with a brain tumor and her experience at The Mayo.

Another friend set up a GoFundMe page and shared it across social media to help pay for medical related expenses. There were donations from complete strangers. The page raised several thousand dollars, and turned out to be a big help in covering medical and travel expenses that quickly began piling up.

My co-workers banned together and offered to donate vacation time so I could keep getting paid while out for surgery and during recovery.

My wife's co-workers did the same.

My co-workers also put together "Travis Day" at the office. They had clients and staff donate all sorts of things and put them up on a silent auction. All of the proceeds were donated to my family. Again, several thousand dollars that turned out to be a huge blessing.

We have received text messages, Facebook messages,

letters, and phone calls - all of them telling us that we're being prayed for and offering to help in any way they could.

These are just a handful of examples of the literally hundreds of stories I could tell about how people around us, some complete strangers, banded together to help us out in our time of need.

The Power of Prayer and Positive Thinking

Regardless of your thoughts on prayer and higher powers, I know for a fact it's good for the soul. Prayer and positivity work wonders at keeping the human spirit alive and kicking. Going through all of this has only verified that for me.

My friends and family from across the country have given their kind words and told me they're praying for us

My wife's boss had my name added to a 24-hour prayer board where people sign up for an hour of the day and promise to pray for those on the list during that hour.

A woman I have never met approached me at church and told me she's a friend of my mom's. She and her husband pray for us every night.

Another friend from across the country sent me a Facebook message. He told me that my family is the topic of his nightly prayers with his wife for that evening.

A member of our church posted that we've been added to the prayer list that circulates the congregation.

Again, these are just a handful of examples of the literally hundreds of prayer stories I could tell. It's a peaceful and humbling thought to know that people I've never met are speaking to God on my behalf. All of this happened in the weeks following our Facebook announcement.

We didn't ask for any of this kind of support. We weren't looking for it when we posted the news on Facebook. All we wanted to do was let our friends and family know what was going on. For the first few days, we kept telling people, "No, you don't have to do that. It's okay. We'll get by … No really, we appreciate it, thank you – but you don't need to do anything!"

Our dismissals fell on deaf ears.

The next week, I went back to work in a vain attempt to return to life as normal until my surgery. A good friend gave me some advice, "In times like these, you just need to be humble and accept the blessings as they're offered." He was right.

Learning to be Humble

Humility is a strange thing. When most people think about being humble, they think about making sure other people take credit over themselves. Don't be boastful or arrogant. Help others and pay it forward. Those are all good things - great things in fact. However, being humble has another side to it. It's this other side of humility my wife and I have found most difficult to grasp.

This side of humility is about accepting help when offered. We've had to force ourselves to put aside our pride and lower the shields. You see, it's not like we were in dire straits to pay our bills, find childcare, or cook meals. "We'll be fine. We'll get by. It'll be okay!"

That's what we kept telling people and that's why it's so difficult to accept the blessings we were being offered. But, we learned to be humble.

It's not like we weren't expecting people to offer help, support and prayers. With this kind of news, you know that's going to happen. It's the sheer volume, the flood of everything, which has completely overwhelmed us. We're more grateful than we can possibly express. The list of thank you cards we sent out kept growing faster and faster! It was almost impossible to keep up. Even then, a thank you card felt miniscule as a way to express our gratitude.

Someday, when we're on the other side of the fence, we're going to pay it forward. Not because we owe anybody or to make up for all the good we've received. We'll do it for the same reason our friends and family have reached out to us: because we're honored to do it.

After dealing with everything that happened the first few weeks after the initial MRI, I had found that I was peaceful about it, even though we didn't actually know anything yet. As my middle daughter, Tatum, put it, "Daddy just has a bump in his head."

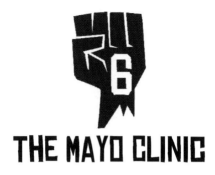

THE MAYO CLINIC

If you haven't heard of the Mayo Clinic, you probably live under a rock. It's one of the best hospitals in the world. Its original location is in Rochester, MN. Since then, they've opened clinics in Florida and Arizona. In fact, in 2014, it was voted #1 in the country for Neurology and Neurosurgery, the exact departments I was being treated in. Here it was in our backyard, only 2 ½ hours from our house in Sauk Rapids.

Our appointments were set for July 10th and 11th of 2014. The first with a neurologist named Dr. Lachance. The second was with a neurosurgeon who would do the actual surgery. His name was Dr. Meyer. He was the Chair of the Neurosurgery Department, making him, at least in my mind, one of the best brain surgeons in the world. Lucky me!

We found out that none of the records or MRI images I had released were sent down. Dr. Lachance didn't have much to go on for my exam. He did a neurological exam, which came back normal.

The neurological exam had me do various exercises to stimulate the brain. Some of them were tapping my feet as fast as possible, looking straight ahead and use my peripheral vision to tell him which of his fingers was moving, etc. He also looked into my eyes for any signs of something wrong with my brain. I responded normally to all of those tests, indicating even further that the tumor was low grade, not fast growing, and that we found it early.

The tumor was in the part of my brain that controls speech and movement; the "Supplemental Motor Area" or SMA for short. It's no wonder I was having thoughts about what people were saying during my seizures. As far as why I would make them swear in my head, I don't know.

That part of the brain actually *initiates* speech and movement. It doesn't do the actual moving. Once movement is initiated, another part of the brain takes over. The brain functions in mysterious ways, but ultimately it worked out for my better interest.

It's weird calling them seizures, which is medically what they are. Technically, they're "partial complex seizures," but I prefer the term "episode." When most people think of a seizure, they think of someone flopping around on the ground with their tongue hanging out. As I learned, there are many kinds of seizures. Only grand mal seizures include uncontrollable muscle spasms.

It's amazing how much I've learned about my brain through this cancer journey.

Dr. Lachance also believed, based on the description of the MRI paper report we had, that it was a moderate-sized infiltrating low-grade glioma. Following his exam, we made several frantic calls to the hospital back home to get the MRI images and medical records sent down right away. Everyone we spoke with was very helpful and apologetic. They got everything sent quickly so we were able to keep the appointment we had the following day with the neurosurgeon.

After we left the first appointment, Kayleigh and I were positive. All the tests came back normal, and it sounded like everything was going to be okay.

We were both famished. In an effort to find some food, and to take our minds off the events of the day, we found a local joint called Newt's. They had amazing burgers and a great beer selection. When I say amazing, I'm not kidding. World class burgers can be found there. And no, they didn't pay me to say that. That place has become a regular stop for us on our trips to Rochester.

The next day, July 11th, we met with the surgeon and his nurse practioner, Nealy Cray. He had the MRI images by then so we were able to look at them together:

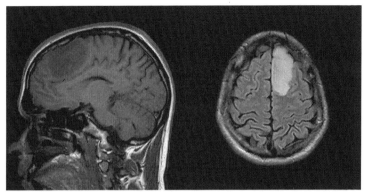

You can see the tumor clearly here. I was told it's about the size of a woman's fist. The first photo shows just how deep into my brain the tumor was growing. It's amazing I didn't have any other side effects.

Dr. Meyer explained how the procedure would go.

"It takes about five hours. Once you're asleep, we'll do a craniotomy. Do you know what that is?"

"No, but it sounds painful!" I jokingly replied.

"Well, you'll be asleep," he joked. "A craniotomy is how we access the brain. We use a surgical saw to cut a small hole in the skull. Once it is removed, we set it aside to be reattached later."

"Once we have access to the tumor," he continued, "we start taking it out little by little so we don't disrupt any part of the brain. Because of how tumors grow, we can't consider this procedure curative. We'll get about 98% of it out and do a biopsy on it. The results of the biopsy will determine what type of tumor it is and will guide your treatment plan after the surgery. Do you have any questions?"

"Yeah," I replied, "what happens if we don't do anything? If we just leave it alone?"

"Well," Dr. Meyer started, "you'll live for two to three years tops."

"Wow!" I was surprised at the short time frame, "this thing has to come out then!"

Dr. Meyer nodded with agreement. "Anything else?"

"Yes. A few things actually," I replied. "What sort of side effects can I expect from this?"

"Given the location of the tumor and the parts of the brain we're operating on, the most common side effect would be loss of speech immediately following surgery. There might be some short term memory loss, trouble with word finding and forming complex sentences."

"It is also possible that you'll have some right-sided weakness," Dr. Meyer went on. "Since the tumor is on the left side of the brain, which controls the right side of the body, those could range from not being able to move your right side at all, to having some difficulty walking, chewing, moving your fingers and toes, lifting your right arm or leg."

"Okay..." I inquired slowly. "What are the chances that any of these will be permanent?"

"I'd say there is well under a 15 percent chance of having permanent side effects."

My wife sat beside me taking notes like crazy; her pen a blur. I was leaning forward in my chair, listening intently. "So, assuming they aren't permanent, how long do the most common side effects typically last?"

"It varies from patient to patient," Dr. Meyer explained. "Some don't have any side effects, others have them for a few hours. But I've seen them last for weeks or months. There really isn't a good way to tell what side effect you'll have or how long they'll last."

"Okay," I replied, somewhat disappointed with the lack of clarity in his answer. I knew he was right though. Everyone is different and there's no way to predict what each individual will do.

"There is one other thing," Dr. Meyer injected.

I perked up.

"Given the location of the tumor, there is a slight chance we'll have to do the surgery while you're awake."

Awake!? I almost shat myself. Good thing I wasn't taking a sip of coffee in that particular moment. It would have ended up all over Dr. Meyer. There's no way in hell I'm having brain surgery awake. I managed to pull myself together and asked why.

"Well," he explained, "since the tumor is in the spot which affects your speech and movement, we'll need to do a Functional MRI before the surgery. Have you ever had one of those before?"

"No."

"It's just like a regular MRI, except they have you do various tasks during the scan, like tapping your fingers in a pattern, counting to yourself, identifying words that rhyme, colors, and a few other things. This will stimulate the parts of the brain for speech and movement and light them up in the MRI pictures."

"Once we see where those areas are in relation to the tumor," he continued, "we can determine if you need to be awake for the surgery."

I was terrified. "Alright," I nervously replied. "Sounds good. Here's to not having to be awake during brain surgery!"

Everyone laughed.

"Anything else?" asked Dr. Meyer.

"No, I think we're good."

"Okay. I'll leave you with Nealy to schedule the surgery and Functional MRI." He shook mine and my wife's hands, then got up and left.

We chose August 7th for the surgery date; just under a month away.

After the Mayo visit in early July, I went home and returned to work, attempting to live life as normal. Every day I'd look at the calendar and count down the days until brain surgery.

Surprisingly, I was calm about the whole thing. Not that I didn't think about it several times a day; I just wasn't debilitated with fear or anxiety. I was at peace. I was in good hands at the Mayo and I was confident the tumor would turn out to be low grade. I'd take some time to recover, and then return to life as usual.

Or so I thought.

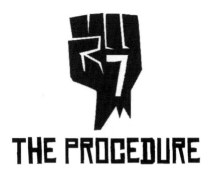

THE PROCEDURE

I have an aunt and uncle, Candy and Greg, who live about an hour north of Rochester in a suburb of the Twin Cities. They offered to let us stay at their place to avoid having to pay for a hotel. We pulled into their driveway on Monday, August 4th.

Candy and Greg hosted Easter every year at their house. To this day, they still host it. Candy is one of my mom's nine siblings. Mom's family has ten children, eight of whom are girls. As you can imagine, family gatherings are large and loud!

There's a long-running joke in our family about my mom and her sisters all having "The Lundborg Laugh." Lundborg is Mom's maiden name. It's not really a laugh so much as it is a cackle. When Mom's sisters are gathered together, there's no hiding it. You can hear them laugh from miles away, and you can pick it out in a crowd of people. If I ever needed to find Mom in a crowd, I just had to listen for The Lundborg Laugh.

When I was a kid, we would drive to Candy and Greg's house the night before Easter to decorate eggs for the big hunt the next day with all of my cousins. They had a big sectional couch. We could rearrange the sections into a circle for someone to sleep on. My siblings and I slept on the sectional-circle when we were younger. We'd watch *Star Wars* every year before going to sleep.

Candy and Greg still had that couch. When we arrived with our girls before surgery, Candy had it setup just like we used to do. I stood there and looked at it for a moment, reminiscing. I took a picture and uploaded it to Facebook, tagging my brother and sister.

I captioned it '*The circle is now complete.*' A pun both of my siblings would understand. I thought it was fitting. If you don't get it, you're not a true *Star Wars* fan.

Uncle Greg passed away in June of 2015 from prostate cancer. At his funeral, Candy came up to us and gave us a big hug. With tears in her eyes, she spoke softly, "Greg took this for you." It was an emotional day for us. My dad gave the eulogy. There wasn't a dry eye in the room. Greg was great man with a gently spirit. His biker look was just a façade. He was a teddy bear at heart, and he adored his nieces and nephews. Especially the little ones.

For a few months after he passed away, Tatum would randomly say, "I miss Uncle Greg." It was sweet and sad at the same time

Our girls stayed with Candy and Greg while we made day trips to Rochester for the Functional MRI and other appointments. We stayed the nights of August 4th and 5th.

We arrived in Rochester on August 5th, a Tuesday. My Functional MRI (fMRI) was that day. It took several hours before I was done. Once I was called back, I had to sit through fMRI training with one of their techs. He ran through each test they'd do and I practiced doing it with him. We did each one a few times before he signed off that I was ready for the actual fMRI.

They also put little black dots on my head with a Sharpie. Eight of them to be exact. The dots were needed during the fMRI to pinpoint exactly where in my brain the movement and speech faculties were located. They needed to be on my face for surgery. Without the dots, Dr. Meyer would be cutting blind. I had to wear them on my face for the next two days.

They were covered in tape while we were in Rochester for the day. When we arrived back at Candy and Greg's house for the night, Kayleigh took maniacal pleasure to color them in with *permanent* marker.

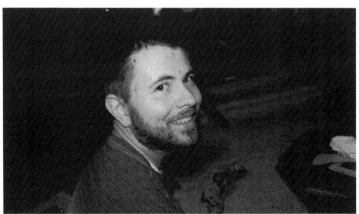

The black Sharpie dots on my face. I had to walk around like this for two days. Good thing I'm not easily embarrassed.

Alexis drew a picture of me with my black dots. We had fun with it. What else is there to do when you have black dots all over your face?

I also had an MRI done for a study I was asked to participate in. This was done free of charge since I was asked to participate in the study. They were testing whether small vibrations would make tumors show up better during an MRI Scan.

In the machine, my head was on a rubber pillow. This pillow would quickly inflate and deflate, inflate and deflate, inflate and deflate; making my head vibrate very rapidly.

"We've never had this cause a seizure in anyone," explained the lady who was running the experiment. That was my biggest concern, now relieved.

"If we have anything worthwhile," she continued, "it'll be available for your surgery on the seventh."

We headed back to Candy and Greg's for another night.

The next morning, we packed our bags and took the girls to Rochester.

On August 6th, the day before my surgery, our families arrived. Kayleigh's parents and youngest sister, my parents, and my siblings all came to support me. We checked into a hotel just a couple of blocks from the hospital.

We all went to Newt's that evening for a "pre-surgery last supper." I made sure to ask Dr. Meyer if I could drink beer before surgery when we met back in July. "Of course!" he replied. "Just don't overdo it." I enjoyed a couple craft brews with supper. I wasn't supposed to eat or drink anything else after 10 p.m.

We enjoyed ourselves. We laughed, told jokes, and tried to keep our minds away from what was coming the next day.

Despite the depressing aura in the air, we all had a good time.

After dinner, I called the hospital to get my check-in time for surgery. The best way to explain what came next is to share my journal entry from that night.

Its 10 p.m. the night before my surgery to remove a brain tumor. I am to check-in at 6 a.m. tomorrow. Surgery should be underway in the 8 a.m. hour. Oddly enough, the last several weeks since we found out have been rather normal.

Aside from the breakdown the night we found out, I have been peaceful about it all. Having no signs or symptoms in that time certainly helped, but I take the peace to be some sort of sign. A sign that it'll be alright and this speed bump will soon be over.

Ever since the surgery date was set, I've been mentally counting down. Four weeks. Two weeks. 1 week. 5 days. 2 days. 24 hours. 12 hours. Just a few minutes ago, I set the alarm on my phone. "6 hours, 27 minutes," it alerted me until the pending wake-up alarm. Then the walk down to the hospital.

There has been an ever-present pit in my stomach for some time now, but nothing debilitating or earth shatteringly nerve wracking. It's there. I'd be lying if I said it wasn't. I'm frightened of the unknown. I worry about my family in case the unthinkable happens. That hasn't consumed my thoughts though. I won't let it.

Being positive, cracking jokes, laughing and living just comes easier, more naturally for me than being down in the dumps.

Tatum isn't sure what to think. She told me tonight that she's nervous, but I don't think she really knows what's going on or what it means.

I think Alexis is more scared than she is willing to let on. Deep down, I think she's afraid I have cancer, which might be the case, but we don't know yet. She puts on a strong face.

My biggest fear about Harper is that she won't remember her daddy in case something happens to me.

As for Kayleigh...she's a trooper. I don't know how I'd get through this without her. Not a chance. Her way of coping is by planning. She has every minute, even silly details thought through and figured out. Right down to packing lists and travel expense reports for the insurance company. It's amazing. She's amazing. I love her more than life itself.

I'm not sure what tomorrow will bring, but I want her with me for all of it.

Brain Surgery

August 7th, 2014, was the first day of the rest of my life. I entered the hospital room with nothing but a bandage around my head and a gown around my waist. I was relieved and frightened all at once. I had never experienced this kind of thing before. A brain tumor had just been extracted from my noggin and here I lay, awake and breathing in a hospital room not more than 24 hours later.

Our alarm went off at 5 a.m. that day. The big girls were sleeping with my parents across the hall, so we only had Harper in our room with us. She slept all night, which was a rarity for her. I wonder if she could sense something major was about to happen?

We got showered and dressed. Most of the time spent in silence. We both knew what the other was thinking about, so there was no sense in asking. Around 5:40, we finished packing our things, put the baby in her stroller and headed for St. Mary's Hospital, just two blocks from our hotel. The sun was just breaking the horizon as we walked the empty streets in silence. Harper fell back to sleep in her stroller. It was eerie and peaceful at the same time. I took my hand out of my pocket and grazed my wife's fingers with mine. She took my hand and squeezed gently. That gentle squeeze was our only communication during the short walk.

The first 24-36 hours are rather a blur in my head, but I do remember bits and pieces.

The check-in line for surgeries was a herd of people. I was surprised it was so busy at 6:00 a.m. There were a handful of lines each leading up to a desk with a clerk behind a computer. Kayleigh took the baby and found a chair nearby while I waited in the shortest line.

Once I was checked-in, I was given a wristband and we waited in the lobby on the main floor of St. Mary's Hospital. Every now and then, someone from the Mayo Clinic would appear through big double doors and call out a group of people. They'd follow the staffer back to the pre-op area.

We were finally called with a group of people. As we walked through the labyrinth of hallways, we made stops at various areas for patients to go to their respective surgeries and procedures. We finally ended up in my area. There were a few others with us from the group. I had no idea where we were. We'd gone up an elevator and meandered through winding hallways. The area we were in had dozens of small rooms for people to get dressed for surgery. Those who came from our group each split off to find their own room.

They had one ready for me, too. It was barely large enough for me, my wife, and the stroller. I was instructed to strip down and put on a hospital gown.

After I was done changing, a nurse came in and verified who I was and why I was there. He scanned my wristband and then asked me to verbally say who I was.

"My name is Travis McGinnis. I'm here for brain surgery," I explained.

"Which side of your brain are we operating on today?" he asked.

I pointed to my left side. He marked the spot on my head with a Sharpie.

"Very good!" he proclaimed as he stood up and left.

It was then we were told that our families wouldn't have a chance to see me until after surgery. I frantically texted my parents while Kayleigh texted hers. I found out later they were just sitting down for breakfast in the hotel lobby. Upon reading our text messages, they dropped their forks and left their meals on the table. They rushed to the hospital so they could see me before I went under the knife.

They made it. My parents, my brother, my sister, and mother-in-law were all there. Our girls were back at the hotel with Kayleigh's dad and sister.

I went around and gave everyone a hug. Dad had tears in his eyes. My sister was crying. My brother was silent, but the look on his face told me everything. My mom and Kayleigh's mom started crying.

"Sorry! We're moms! This is what we do!" Kayleigh's mom, Connie, joked. We all forced an awkward laugh.

My mom held me tight. I could hear her sobbing into my shoulder. This could very well be the last time she saw me.

Last but not least, I hugged my wife.

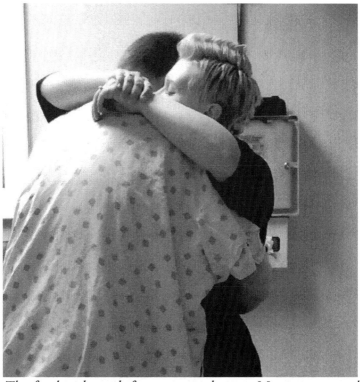

The final embrace before we parted ways. My sister snapped this shot, unbeknownst to us. It has become one of my favorite pictures. They say a picture is worth a thousand words. They're right.

There was a gurney waiting for me. I climbed in and my wife snapped one last photo:

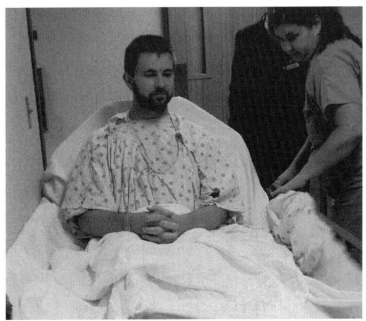

This was taken just seconds before I left my wife and family behind. You can see the black dots on my face to guide the surgeon. I was in contemplative silence. I just said what could possibly have been my final goodbyes to my family.

I was wheeled down the hall and into a dark alcove. Pre-op. I was alone. Cold. Nervous. My whole body was shaking. My teeth were chattering uncontrollably. Another nurse came in to, again, verify who I was and why I was there. After scanning my wristband, he asked me the same questions as before. He left when he was done, and I was again alone.

It felt like an eternity, but the clock on the wall showed

seven minutes had passed. I knew they'd be putting IV's in, so I tucked my icy hands under my body to warm them; IV's go in better when the veins are warm.

Next, a doctor comes into my dark alcove. He shook my hand and identified himself as Dr. Anderson with anesthesiology. He told me he'd be the one putting me under for my surgery and would be in the room the whole time monitoring my vitals. He also did the same song and dance as the previous nurse. Who are you and why are you here? Then he left to prep for my surgery.

Another eternity passed.

Finally, a gentleman approached my gurney to wheel me to the operating theater. He asked the same questions as the first two visitors; I guess they can't be too cautious when it comes to brain surgery. He was short, stalky, had a ponytail, and a graying beard. He looked uncannily like Uncle Greg. So much so, I did a double take just to make sure I wasn't seeing things. His smile lit up the dark room. He looked as if he'd be more comfortable in a tattered pair of jeans and a Harley T-shirt than in hospital scrubs.

The journey to the operating room was a maze of hallways. At least, that's how I remember it. I made small talk with Gray Beard to ease my nerves. Just the presence of a familiar face, even though we had never met, was calming.

As we approached our destination, our conversation turned to the task at hand: removing a tumor from my head.

"They're going to come at you like a herd," Gray Beard added as we wheeled into the O.R.

I was placed onto a table and, as warned, had all sorts of people approach me from all different angles.

The operating room was brightly lit with light yellow walls. There was a window looking out into the hallway; I assumed for family members to watch. Or perhaps, it was for medical students so they can take notes to learn during a live surgery. I'm not sure; I never asked. My family had to sit in the waiting room the whole time, so I never found out what the window was for.

There were four large, flat-screen televisions about ten feet up on the wall. Three were right next to each other and the fourth was on top of the middle one. The bottom three had pictures of my MRI where the tumor was located, and the one on top had what appeared to be vital statistics to monitor during surgery.

"You're going to feel a stick in your hand," said Gray Beard. It was the needle for the IV. It hurt; not a lot, but enough to feel the pain shoot up my arm.

I lost track of who was in the room with me. First, Dr. Meyer came in, shook my hand, and asked me some simple questions. Then one of his aids came in.

While he was talking, Dr. Meyer stifled a cough with his fist. He was wearing a surgical mask. *That's not very sanitary!* I thought. It quickly left my mind. After all, he was Chair of the Neurosurgery Department for the Mayo Clinic. He's basically the best brain surgeon in the world. And I was lucky enough to have him operate on me. They both disappeared, presumably to scrub up for surgery.

Next, Dr. Anderson with anesthesiology made his appearance. "Long time no see!" he joked. I was too scared to respond. I just laid there. Silently trembling.

"You're going to feel a burn go up into your right arm," Dr. Anderson explained. "It means you'll soon be taking a nap."

I felt the burn. The bright lights overhead began to fade away as I slipped into a deep sleep.

Beeping. That's the next thing I remember.

I was waking up.

Nearly five hours had passed. The procedure was complete.

I saw bright lights as I opened my eyes. I wasn't in the same room as before. Everything was blurry. I closed my eyes again.

"Travis, can you hear me?" asked an unfamiliar voice. I thought it was in my head as I slipped in and out of consciousness. It was Nealy Cray, Dr. Meyer's nurse practitioner. She was behind a surgical mask, so I didn't recognize her at first.

Nauseated, I vomited. I later learned that I had puked half a dozen times already. Apparently, it's possible to throw up when you're unconscious. Who knew?

I felt sick to my stomach. I puked again into a blue bowl. I remember little details like that. The beeping sound, Nealy's voice, the color of the bowl. The remaining contents of my stomach came up that time. The rest after that were nothing but dry heaves.

Whenever I puked, sneezed, yawned, or my head suddenly jerked around, I could feel and *hear* the fluid sloshing around the hole in my brain where the tumor used to live. It's a difficult sensation to describe; like hearing something while you're underwater, but I wasn't underwater. It was so weird.

I'm not sure how long it took that hole to fill with fluid, but it was several weeks after the surgery before the sloshing finally stopped.

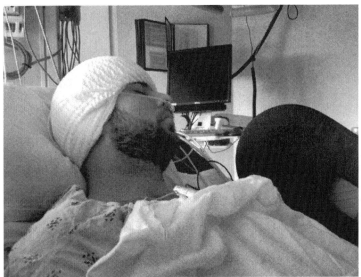

I was passed out in the ICU. I'm not sure when this was taken. You can see my unshaven face. It would continue to grow for the next two days.

I was unable to speak. Mute. I remember trying to speak while waking up, but nothing came out. I couldn't even grunt or groan. My voice box was down for the count. I was incapable of producing any sounds whatsoever. It was a side effect of having my brain cut open. I was told that would be a possibility, but deep down, I hoped it wouldn't happen. I was terrified that my speech would never come back, that I'd never be able to talk again.

There are so many things we take for granted every day. Our ability to speak and communicate with other people is what separates us from animals. I lost that ability, and it was terrifying.

"Do you want me to get your wife?" Nealy asked gently. Unable to speak, I nodded instead.

"Hi, Baby," was the next thing I remember hearing. It was the soft voice of my wife. I looked up at her, smiled, and then passed back out.

The next blur of visitors was rather fuzzy, but I remember them in order. I was in and out of consciousness between the sets of visitors. First, Mom and Dad. Dad touched my foot. I felt squeezes on my hands. I'm not sure how long they were around.

Next to visit were my brother and sister. I'm not sure how much time had passed from after Mom and Dad left to when they showed up. I assume it wasn't very long. I remember hearing them ask things and me nodding to them, but not much else.

Then, my aunt, Mary Pat; and mother-in-law, Connie came in. I remember looking up to see Mary Pat on my left and Connie on my right. I closed my eyes and passed back out.

The next thing I remember is seeing my lovely wife's smiling face. I'm not sure how long I had been out.

The nurse asked me something; I'm not sure what it was. I tried so hard to speak. My brain struggled to connect the dots that turn thoughts into speech. After what felt like an eternity, I spoke for the first time in probably 18 hours.

"Ugh. I'm good," I groaned.

The smile on my bride's face was from ear to ear. She heard me talk!

August 7ᵗʰ
(This is from Kayleigh's journal while I was in surgery.)

It has been a long day of waiting. Travis got to the pre-surgery area, and we found out we wouldn't be able to see him until after the surgery. Mike, Ada, Aaron, Kayla and my mom left their plates at the hotel and ran over. They got here just in time for hugs and kisses.

It was kind of surreal to leave him there, but the support was nice. Harper was such a great baby! She slept through the night and then some! She made friends and helped to pass the time.

Surgery finally got under way at 9:21 a.m. and the resection began around 11 a.m. The surgery went faster than the anticipated five hours. They called about four hours after the start to have me come down to talk with Dr. Meyer. Longest elevator ride ever!

Dr. Meyer was full of good news! The surgery went just as planned. They removed the tumor (except for the microscopic fingers), about 98% in all. It was the size of Nealy's fist! That area is now filled with fluid.

Nealy came to talk with me while we were still in the visitor's lounge. She told me that Travis could move all of his muscle groups but that he was mute, unable to talk. He wanted to, but couldn't get the words out. She said he was very frustrated! She also wanted me to know that with his inability to speak, a lot of his facial expression was lacking. He had a flat affect. She also said he was very nauseated, which is why he was still in the PACU.

After I got the news and shed a few tears (this was one of Travis' fears going into surgery), I went to the other side of the waiting room wall to tell the others.

The phone finally rang in the waiting room.

My mom grabbed it and gave it to me. The nurse said he was in his room and we could go see him. I went in first, as Travis said that was what he wanted, and I did too. My heart broke to see my tough hubby all bandaged up, lying in his bed. I'm not sure which was harder to see...him unable to talk to me or the lack of emotion on his face. I just leaned on the rail of the bed and took his hand. He squeezed my fingers and I told him I loved him.

After a while, I asked him if I should bring his family in. He nodded. I left to get Mike and Ada. I made it to the hallway before silent tears fell down my cheeks. I worked to control myself before I reached the waiting room.

Before bringing Travis' parents back, I tried to prepare them. When we got to Travis' room, they took turns rubbing his shoulder and quietly letting him know they were there. He was still so out of it and so tired.

Next his siblings came in, and then my mom and Mary Pat, Travis' aunt.

As I walked them out, Mary Pat gave me a hug and told me how blessed Travis was to have me. I cried and thanked her...all I thought about was how blessed Travis and I were to have each other and our beautiful girls.

I asked Travis if he wanted me to stay in the ICU with him and he nodded yes. I ran to get stuff at the hotel. While I was there, I took the girls aside and told them about Daddy. I told them he was fine, that he could move everything but still couldn't talk. Tatum quietly said, "Okay." Alexis asked me if Daddy is going to die. I told her everyone dies, but Daddy is not going to die right now. She seemed very relieved.

Back at the hospital, I sat and held Travis' hand for a long time, then laid down.

At about 11 p.m. he was getting restless. The nurse and I were helping him get more comfortable. Then he spoke. "Uh...I'm good." The nurse and I exchanged excited looks and she told him it was nice to hear him finally talk! I was so excited to hear those words! I'm sure my grin was huge! The rest of the night was pretty uneventful.

I was in the ICU for about a day. I was visited by Dr. Meyer's staff and aides. There were so many of them, I can't remember their names. They were testing for any side effects from the surgery, and they found quite a few.

Most notably, I was unable to speak for the first 18 hours or so afterwards. Once that came back, by biggest struggle was with thinking and forming thoughts, and then turning those thoughts into words. At least I didn't any get headaches from trying.

August 8th - Friday

Another very busy day! Dr. Shepard, one of Dr. Meyer's aides, came in with another resident to see how I was doing. They were impressed with my progress.

"You're too healthy to be in the ICU!" Dr. Shepard exclaimed.

They transferred me to the Neuro Floor, out of intensive care. They also removed the bandage from my head and checked the incision, which was sealed up with about a million staples. It looked good. Dr. Meyer did a fine job.

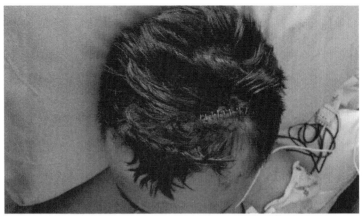

My gnarly incision after surgery. After seeing this, it's amazing I actually survived after having my brain cut open!

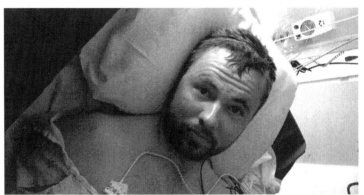

Laying in the ICU after the bandage was removed. This is my "Really? Must you?" look.

Dr. Shepard and his assistant checked my right side and did a few tests. My right side worked, but was not as fast or as coordinated as my left side. They instructed me to move my left foot back and forth as fast as I could. I did so with ease. Then it was the right foot's turn. It was slow. Sluggish. Deliberate. Uncoordinated.

Not being able to control my limbs was so irritating and frustrating. I could do it just fine 24 hours ago, but now? Nope. Nothing.

After they left, Nealy came in and was excited to see my speech back already.

Then, some folks from Physical/Occupational and Speech Therapy came in to do an assessment. For speech, they advised waiting a week or two before deciding to take speech therapy back home.

"A lot can improve over a couple weeks," I was told. "That will also give time for the swelling of your brain to go down, which can have a big impact on speech issues."

I kept using the same words and phrases over and over again. My vocabulary was quite limited. My go-to response to most things was, "Correct."

I said it all the damn time. I said it so much that even I got annoyed with myself. I'd vow to use a different word, and then I'd say it again, because that's the only word I could think of. Correct. Correct. Correct.

I'd even say it when it wasn't the appropriate answer to a question.

"How are you feeling today, Mr. McGinnis?" one of the nurses asked.

"Correct." I responded. She gave me the *try again* look. I'm sure she hears those kind of things all the time on the neuro floor. Every patient up there has issues with their brain.

Once I realized my error, which happened more often than not, I changed my response. "I'm pretty good, all things considered," or something to that effect.

"That's more like it!" she'd reply with a smile.

My wife smiled too. She was more patient with me than I was, though she admitted once I was over the whole "correct" phase, that she was getting rather irritated by it as well.

At about 2 p.m. that day, we prepped to have me moved up to my new room, out of the ICU. By prep, I mean they pulled out the catheter that was inserted while I was in surgery and ripped off the monitors from my chest.

Neither of those were pleasant. Not one little bit. First was the catheter.

"Turn your head and cough," one of the nurses instructed as she was getting ready to deflate the bag in my bladder. I didn't think people actually used that phrase in real life; I thought it was just from comedy television.

I turned my head. I coughed. She pulled.

The cough and the pull didn't line up. It stung. It burned. My body contorted on my bed. I winced and slowly shuddered out an exhale in painful agony. That's not an experience I care to ever have again.

"You might feel some urgency to use the bathroom," the nurse continued after the catheter had been removed. There was blood on it. I looked down. There was blood *down there* too.

"You also might see some blood in your urine the first couple of times. That's normal." I was relieved to have the catheter ordeal over, and to know that blood was normal. That's not a part of my body I want to have abnormal things happening to!

Next, it was time for the six monitoring patches on my chest and stomach to come off. The ones on my stomach weren't too bad since there wasn't much hair. The ones on my chest? That's another story. Ever see *The 40 Year Old Virgin*? Remember the chest waxing scene? It was a lot like that. Only worse. Slow or fast didn't matter. Either way, it hurt like hell. I had bald spots on my chest for weeks afterwards. I bit my lip, squeezed my eyes tight, and shrugged my shoulders into my ears to prepare for the onslaught.

Once the chest monitor removal agony was over, I got into a wheel chair as my wife gathered my things. We made our way to the neurology floor, one level above us.

I was capable of walking, but was not very steady on my feet. We would practice that in my new room and at the hotel when we were discharged.

Once we got to my room, which actually had a shower in it, I promptly stripped down and jumped – not literally – right in. I felt gross. I looked gross. I was washing dried blood out of my incision for weeks afterwards. It's amazing how much gets under the staples and into your hair. I think it was nearly two months later when I saw the last flake of dried blood wash down the drain.

Kayleigh helped with my shower. She didn't want me alone in there because I was so unsteady on my feet. They had a chair I could sit on and she washed my hair the best she could. I put on a clean hospital gown and a fresh application of deodorant. My face needed a good shave, but that would have to wait until we were discharged. I would have to deal with looking like Grizzly Adams for a few more days.

My kids were dying to see their daddy, but they weren't allowed in the ICU. They hadn't seen me in almost two days. They were so cute when they came in. Tatum crawled up in my bed and claimed her spot on my lap right away.

They were excited to tell me about their adventures with Grandpa and Auntie around Rochester while I was in surgery. They were also excited I was able to talk again. They were expecting me to be unable to speak, since that's the last Kayleigh had told them.

Kayleigh was overjoyed to see me with my girls. It was so much easier for me to interact with them than with other adults. It was probably because their minds are less complex, simpler. My brain at the time was just better suited to interact with children.

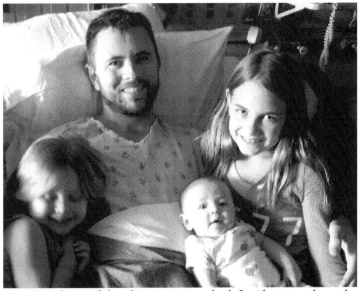

My three beautiful girls. Tatum on the left, Alexis on the right, Harper on my lap.

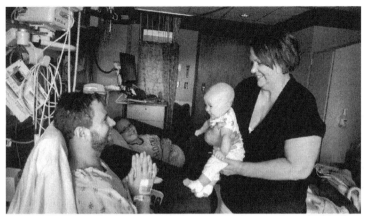

Me playing with Harper while my mother-in-law holds her. My sister, Kayla, is laying on the chair in the background.

After the girls visit, I wanted to get some rest. Everyone went to the Canadian Honker Restaurant for dinner and then back to the hotel. Kayleigh came back to the hospital for another night with me. We sat in our chairs since I was finally allowed to get out of bed. We watched Shawshank Redemption on TV. It was nice and relaxing to share that moment with my bride. We had a busy day, so it felt good to have some time to ourselves. We held hands, and made small talk as best as I could manage with my limited vocabulary. Just having her there with me was comforting.

August 9th - Saturday

We had another busy morning. Dr. Shepard came in again and said we could get discharged that afternoon. I know. Discharged two days after brain surgery. Crazy, right?

There was another gentleman on the neuro floor who had brain surgery the same day I did. We didn't meet or anything, but from the looks of it, he wasn't doing nearly as well as I was. I don't think he was moving or talking yet. His wife just sat by him, holding his hand. He was moving somewhat, just not recovering nearly as quickly as I was. I imagine they kept him for a few days longer.

His family sat with mine in the waiting room. We had our surgeries at the same time, and they ended about the same time, too. Kayleigh rode the elevator with his wife up for the initial meeting with the doctors after our respective procedures. They walked together down the long hallway in silence.

It was so weird being discharged from the hospital just two days after brain surgery. That's the most important organ in your body, and they just let me walk out of the hospital two days later. They keep patients who've had open heart surgery for many days, maybe even weeks, after their procedure. Several days are spent just in the ICU. Brain surgery patients? Two days and out.

I had an MRI that morning. While I was down having it done, Dr. Meyer came in and spoke to Kayleigh.

"Travis should make a full recovery!" he told her, "Just keep him walking and talking and it will get easier."

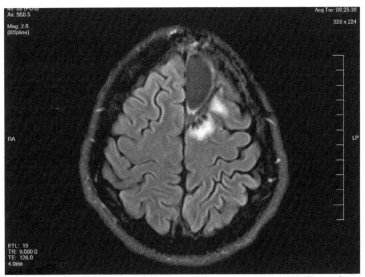

My post-surgery MRI scan. The white areas are swelling from the surgery. I now had a fist-sized hole in my brain.

The folks from Physical and Occupational Therapy prescribed me a few exercises to restore my right side coordination and strength. One of them was to loosen and tighten a nut onto a bolt. So, my dad and brother took a trip to the hardware store and picked up several bolts and nuts of varying sizes for me to work with.

The point of this exercise is to fine tune the small motor movements in my fingers.

Also that morning, before discharge, the same group of doctors from the day before showed up again to do more tests. One of them had me look at an inked drawing. In it was a mother standing at the sink doing dishes. She was wearing an apron. The sink was spilling over onto the floor. The doctor pointed to the sink and asked me to describe what I saw.

I thought hard about it. Not because I didn't know what to say, but because I couldn't think of the right word. I knew that I knew the word; I just couldn't think of it. It was infuriating! After a few moments, I gave up.

"The sink is wet," I struggled. I knew it was wrong, but that was the closest word I could think of. The word I was looking for was *overflowing*. I struggled with word-finding for a long time. To this day, it still happens occasionally, but not nearly as much as the first few weeks following surgery.

Also in the picture was a little boy climbing on a chair to reach a box of cereal in the cupboard. He had a chair leaning against the counter and a box on top of the chair to stand on. It looked precarious and dangerous. There was another child visible outside through the window. He was playing on the tire swing hanging from the backyard tree. The mother at the sink was focused on the child outside. I was asked what I would call this picture. I don't remember exactly what I said, but it was something along the lines of "Boy climbing on chair while mother stands at sink looking into yard." It was a very literal and long-winded way of describing what was going on in the picture verbatim.

They were testing my brain functions to see if I could articulate complex scenarios in simple terms. I failed miserably.

If I were to look at that same picture today, I would just call it "Chaos."

Next, I was asked to explain the metaphor, "Don't count your eggs before they hatch." They wanted to see if I could understand and describe what metaphors are. I knew the phrase, I had heard it before and used it many times myself. I *knew* what it meant, and I told them so. I just wasn't able to *explain* it with words.

They also had me practice writing. That was something I didn't expect to be broken. My handwriting was atrocious. When I look back at my journal entries from the time, I could barely read my own words. It looked like a three year old had written it.

Then, they asked me to sign my name. That didn't go well either. I butchered my once beautiful autograph. I spent months in 6th grade practicing my signature until I had it down just the way I wanted it. I've been using the same one ever since.

I was asked to write the same things over and over again for practice. "Just keep writing. It'll get better!" they promised.

I wrote my first, middle, and last name. I wrote my address. I signed my name. I wrote my phone number. My wife was looking over my shoulder during this. She inquired about the phone number. "Whose number is that?"

I paused and looked. "Mine?" I sniped as if it was obvious.

"That's not your phone number, Babe," she replied.

I looked again. She was right. It was my parent's old home phone number. The one I had been reciting to people for 20 years. It was so engrained in my memory. It was the first phone number that came to mind when I started writing. The brain is a creature of habit, and habit is what it falls back on when it cannot create something new. This is a lesson I was quickly learning.

That afternoon, we were discharged from the hospital after only two days.

I showered before we left and then changed into my street clothes after they took the IV's out of my hands. I had one in each hand. I could still see the marks on my wrists where they had several more IV's attached during surgery. All but two of the IVs were removed before they woke me up, and I had three small IV scars in the inside of my left wrist that I could see for a few months afterwards.

My dad drove the car up to the front and I was taken out in a wheelchair. Again, just in case my stability wasn't there.

We chose a hotel within walking distance from the hospital, so it was just a short drive. Dad dropped us off at the front door then went to park the car. It was surreal being there. I had just had brain surgery barely two days ago and there I was, standing up and looking around the hotel lobby.

Up in our room, I talked to my girls for a little while and gave them each a stuffed animal as a gift for being so good during our time at the hospital. The girls went back home with Kayleigh's parents that afternoon. My parents opted to stay another night with us.

We kept the baby in our room while my parents were in their room across the hall. They offered to let her stay the night in their room, but we decided to keep her.

We should have taken them up on their offer.

The baby was up several times that night and so was I. When she cried really loud, it would give me a headache. Aside from that, I fortunately, had very minimal pain. These headaches happened for several weeks after surgery, but the only time I would get a headache was when the baby would scream really loudly.

You know the cry. Babies are still only a few months old and they start to scream. Their tongue curls up, tears trickle out of their clenched eyelids, and their faces turn bright red. Those are the screams that gave me headaches.

I was on pain killers for a few days: a tapering dose of Oxycodone plus prescription strength Tylenol as needed. I didn't feel any pain aside from the headaches when the baby would cry really loud. I'm not sure if that was because the drugs were doing their job, or if I just didn't have any pain. I wasn't going to risk the pain by not taking the pills, so down they went.

August 10th - Sunday

The next morning, we met my parents for breakfast in the lobby. They offered to take Miss Harper so we could get my first cup of post-surgery Caribou Coffee. Obviously we agreed because I love Caribou, and lucky for me, it was right next door to the hotel.

We sat outside in the sun, and made small talk. The hardest part for me was just thinking of something to say. I'm usually one of the most talkative people in the room. Being at a loss for words was both scary and irritating as hell for me.

When we got back to the hotel a short while later, my parents offered to take Harper back to their house, while we stayed in Rochester until my neurology appointment, which we still didn't have scheduled. I quickly agreed, though Kayleigh wanted Harper to stay with us as a mental distraction. However, she told me later that day we had made the right decision to send Harper with my parents. We needed to focus on me right now, and not having a baby around made that much easier. Plus, I wouldn't get headaches when she cried and we could both get a decent night's sleep.

After Mom and Dad left with Harper, Kayleigh helped me shower again. She joked about if the crap in my hair would ever come out!

Then, we went in search of dinner. We chose Chipotle because, duh, it's Chipotle. Chipotle is yummy-awesome. It was also next to Target where we got some walking in and picked up some clean clothes, groceries, and shaving supplies to trim down my grisly beard.

We spent the rest of the evening playing cards and watching Shark Week on TV. Oh, Mike Rowe. He's the Discovery Channel mascot.

We also walked up and down the hallway in the hotel. I was doing the walking exercises prescribed by the doctors. Kayleigh was walking along next to me in case I lost my balance. One lady gave us a funny look as she awkwardly walked around us on her way to the elevators.

"I know, we look silly," Kayleigh told her.

"Yeah…you do," she replied, not really sure what to think. Obviously, she had no idea why we were walking goofy in the halls.

I walked forward, walked backwards, grapevine, heel to toe. We did the same thing the night before. My walking and balance had improved considerably in 24 hours.

Back in our room, the big girls called to chat and tell us about their day.

"Mommy, can you guys come home now? I miss you!" Tatum asked in her sad voice. It broke our hearts to have to say no. We both got a little choked up.

We told her to snuggle the stuffed animal I got her whenever she missed us.

Talking to my girls just came naturally to me. It wasn't as difficult or forced. I needed to speak to them in simple terms, which was much easier to say than complex thoughts.

As to be expected whenever you're away from home, life outside of Rochester continued without us. We got a text from Kayleigh's mom. The water heater at our house was out. We had them call a plumber to go look at it. However, my dad didn't trust that company. He has worked in plumbing and heating wholesale for over 30 years; he knows every plumber in the industry. If he doesn't trust someone, I believe him.

So, we had another company come out and take a look, the one my dad recommended. They told us the water heater needed to be replaced. My dad knew the owner, and had told him about my tumor shortly after we found out. When he saw our last name on the work order, he called my dad to inquire if that water heater was for us. He replaced it for free and paid for the water heater out of his own pocket.

The generosity of some people blows me away. I've never met this guy, yet here he was paying for a replacement water heater for a complete stranger. All because he knew it would be a financial burden in this chapter of our lives. We made sure to send that company a thank you note.

While we were in the St. Cloud Hospital right after the first MRI (where they found the tumor), my Jeep broke down. We had the Jeep towed to one of our car dealer clients from work. I later found out that my boss had taken care of the bill.

"How much do we owe you?" I asked him.

"Nothing," he replied, "Don't worry about it. Consider me your personal car care assistant!"

I chuckled and thanked him for his generosity.

I guess being in hospitals is prime time for something major to break because we're not around to do anything about it. It's always something, and they never happen at a convenient time. Though, they wouldn't be problems if they happened at a convenient time, now would they?

August 11th - Monday

We had the same routine again this morning. Kayleigh and I made the short walk from the hotel to Caribou Coffee. It was raining, so we sat inside. I just stared out the window, occasionally glancing at her. I sipped my latte in silence.

"What are you thinking?" she asked.

"I don't know."

"What do you mean?"

"I mean I don't know. I don't know what to say to you, or to anybody. My mind is blank." I spoke very deadpan. My speech affect was still flat and unemotional.

So, we sat in silence drinking our coffees. I enjoyed her presence though. Just being around her made me feel calm, like everything in the world was right.

She asked me to name each of my co-workers' first and last names. I did pretty well. I only missed the last name of our new intern.

Back at the hotel, we tried to get more of the crap out of

my hair. We were gentle around the staples, because we didn't want to incision to open back up. Little by little, though, my head was getting clean! Then, I did some strength exercises and hand exercises with the nuts and bolts.

We bought sandwich supplies at Target the previous day so we wouldn't have to eat out for every meal. We had lunch in the room, took a short nap, and then watched some TV – Shark Week again - until it was time for supper.

We headed to the mall for some more walking and to find a bite to eat. As we were walking around, a towering black man wearing a black and white striped shirt with black pants walked by. He looked like a football referee. I presumed he worked at the sporting goods store in the mall. I leaned into my wife and remarked, "Look! It's Shaq!" I was speaking much louder than I thought, because he heard my comment and looked right at us with "the look."

Apparently, my thought and speech volume filters were also missing after surgery! Kayleigh half-jokingly scolded me, though it was pretty funny. We picked up our pace to avoid any further embarrassment on my part.

We had A&W for supper and then Cold Stone Creamery for dessert. We were both full from supper, but Cold Stone was right there and oh so delicious. We ate ourselves stupid.

We walked the mall for a good hour and I rocked it the whole time, but I was getting tired. We headed back to the hotel.

The girls called us again that night and told us about their day. Alexis had hockey practice and was asked to possibly be a goalie for the tournament that coming weekend. She told us she missed us and was excited for us to come home the next day.

After the phone calls, I found a new pathology report had been posted in my Mayo Clinic App. It was worse than we thought. The tumor was a Grade 3 Oligoastrocytoma.

I read my journal entry from the next day:

I found out yesterday that the tumor in my head is a Stage III Glioma. I'm not sure how that makes me feel. Awful, I guess? It could be worse…could be a stage IV tumor. I'm having a hard time finding the positives. I'm not really sure how to react to something like this, you know? I…

The entry stopped there. It took about twenty minutes to write that short paragraph. My brain struggled the entire time to find the words I wanted to write and to sum up what I was feeling.

We decided not to tell our family until we spoke with Dr. Lachance at our appointment that afternoon. We also agreed to think positive. Much easier said than done. Snuggles, hugs, and kisses helped to ease the immense and overwhelming feelings. I'm so glad Kayleigh was there with me.

Going through this cancer nightmare, I can honestly say I've experienced emotions I've never had before. Others I have had before, but at a completely new level of intensity. They run the gamut from positive to negative, all of them off the charts in terms of intensity and depth.

So, what's my prognosis? How long do I have? How did the meeting with Dr. Lachance go? I'll get to that later.

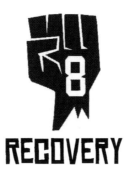

RECOVERY

I spent about six weeks at home recovering from surgery. My speech and handwriting improved exponentially during that time, but I still wasn't as mentally sharp as I was before. It has gotten remarkably better since then, though. To this day, when I'm tired or stressed, I still struggle with complex thoughts and communicating intricate details about a topic. I'm not completely debilitated by it; it just takes me longer to wrap my head around something that once came naturally to me. I hope it gets better. My biggest fear is that I'll never be fully "100% Travis" like I was before. Only time will tell.

About a week after we got home, my coworkers came over in full force with a giant card our Creative Director had designed for me. They all signed it and put a note of encouragement inside. It brought a tear to my eye, and a big ear-to-ear smile on my face, at least that's what I tried to do. My facial expressions were still flat from surgery.

All of Leighton Interactive was there, but the card was signed by nearly every employee at Leighton Enterprises. There were probably 50 signatures on it.

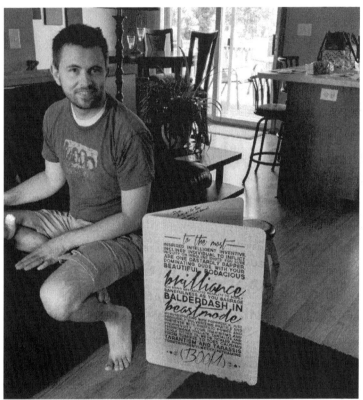

The giant card our Creative Director designed for me. The goofy smile on my face is because my affect was still there. I had trouble making facial expressions for a few weeks.

Our CEO came over as well. He took us all out to lunch at a local pizza joint called House of Pizza. My speech was still sluggish, so I didn't say much. When I did have something to say, I had to think hard about what I wanted to express, rehearse it in my head first, and then speak. That process got much faster and more efficient over the next few weeks. Eventually, my speech returned to normal. Slowly but surely.

I'd occasionally get my words mixed up trying to spit out what I wanted to say. I recall one incident when I was speaking to Tatum. She wanted to have fruit snacks before she finished her supper.

"Tatum, you need to finish your supper before you can have your fruit loops. Ugh…loop fruits…dammit!"

I swore in front of my kids; something I've never done before. I tried to continue my thought, "Snack fru…fruit snacks! That's what I was trying to say!"

All the girls thought it was hilarious. I was just pissed that I couldn't get my words out. I *knew* what I wanted to say. I had the words in my head. It was infuriating that my brain and mouth would not work together to say something so simple.

In the early stages of recovery, I experienced something I never would have expected. I had to re-learn how to do certain things, things I never would have thought about needing to re-learn. Simple things, like how to brew a cup of coffee.

We have a Keurig. I put in a K-Cup, pressed the brew button, and walked away while the machine did its magic.

Then, I heard something strange. It was the sound of coffee brewing into the tray. I forgot to put a cup underneath. Dammit again! Here's the worst part of it. I did the exact same thing the next day.

For the next few days, I had to intentionally think about each step in the process:

Open the machine.
Take out the old K-Cup.
Throw it away.
Put in a new K-Cup.
Close the machine.
Grab a coffee cup from the cupboard.
Place the cup under the brewer.
Press the brew button.

Before the surgery, I had the entire coffee brewing process scripted out in my brain – I never even thought about the steps involved. After surgery, that whole script was missing. I had to re-learn each step. Kayleigh will never let me live it down. She still pokes fun at me for it.

"Don't forget the cup!" she jokes occasionally as I start making a cup of coffee.

I also forgot how to change a diaper. I wish that would have not come back. Then Kayleigh would be stuck with all the dirty diapers.

"Sorry, Babe. I forgot!" It would have been great.

You're probably wondering if it was a wet diaper or poopy diaper when I realized I forgot.

It was a poopy diaper. A massive one.

I could smell Harper from across the room. She was ripe, and ready to be changed. I gave her a few more minutes to finish. You know, just in case.

I picked her up, laid her on the couch, and proceeded to start changing her diaper. It wasn't until I had her pants and diaper off that I realized what I'd forgotten. Two things actually: a new diaper, and the wipes.

By this time, there was poop everywhere. On my hands, on the couch, still on the baby's bottom. Everywhere.

"Kayleigh," I yelled. "Help!"

She came dashing across the house, thinking there was an emergency. She was both appalled and laughing at the same time. I was just confused. How could I forget a diaper and wipes? I've changed so many diapers in my life. That was another script that just went missing. Gone. Vanished without a trace.

Kayleigh did the diaper changing for a while after that. When I felt I was ready, she stood nearby – just in case.

After two weeks, I scheduled an appointment with my family practice provider, Dr. Wyne, to remove the staples from my head. He's the one who ordered the MRI a few months prior. The Mayo gave us a sealed and sanitized staple remover in case they didn't have one.

I was expecting it to hurt, but it really didn't. A few staples pinched a little bit, but that was the extent of it. You'd think that having inch-long staples yanked from your cranium would hurt something fierce. Apparently not.

He asked how I was doing and how the surgery went. He was glad to see I was speaking and, for the most part, back to normal.

I took it easy those next few weeks. I'd get sporadic headaches, but mostly when the baby would scream bloody murder.

Since I wasn't allowed to drive, my wife got to chauffeur

me around. I mostly had her take me to the office to see my colleagues.

I stopped into work to say "Hi!" a few times, but I wouldn't do any actual work because my long term disability had a 90-day waiting period before it kicked in. If I worked at all during that period, I'd have to start the 90-days over again. I sure didn't want that. So, I just made my rounds and visited with co-workers.

They asked how I was doing, and filled me on what I missed while I was out. It was great seeing everyone, regardless of whether I was working. It was tough being away from my job and people I loved, so it was nice being able to at least stop in to chit-chat every now and then.

During that time, I also made an appointment with a speech therapist. She worked with me a few times on my speech and memory. The problems I was experiencing were with expressing very high-level, complicated thoughts. We quickly came to realize it was nothing she could help with. Those issues are difficult to diagnose and to treat because they're so hard to pinpoint other than "something just isn't right." I'd just have to give it time before those high-level thoughts and memory problems took care of themselves. I did have mental exercises to help with those things though.

Radiation was scheduled to begin a little over a month after surgery, on Monday, September 15th.

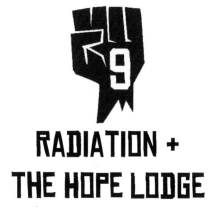

RADIATION +
THE HOPE LODGE

A week before radiation was to begin, we made a trip to Rochester to meet with my radiation oncologist, Dr. Stafford. He was an ex-marine. Big guy. Gentle spirit. During our visit, we went over exactly what radiation was, how it worked and what side effects I could expect along with the chances of each side effect occurring.

The most common ones were hair loss and headaches. Those happen in almost all cases, especially for those patients getting radiation to the head.

Other, less common side effects, are short-term and long-term memory loss. Most times it's not permanent. Another less common side effect is blindness. That one scared me. In fact, going blind is one of my biggest fears. It has been my entire life. I'd rather be deaf and mute than not be able to see. Blindness only happens if they need to radiate near the optic nerve. In my case, we were close, but not close enough for blindness to be a concern.

Another side effect is new tumor growth - usually benign - in the area being treated. Those happen about 1% of the time and typically several years after radiation therapy.

The final, and worst side effect, is brain damage. Which means - you guessed it - death. It happens in so few cases that there isn't a percentage for it. It also tends to happen many years down the road.

During my recovery, while prepping for radiation, we decided to buy a bunch of books for me to read while I was down in Rochester for six weeks.

One of those books was one I'd heard great things about. It has been on my reading list for many years. When we bought it, I kept putting off reading it for some reason. Whenever it was time to pick out a new book to read, I'd look through the books we purchased. I'd look at that book, pull it out, thumb through the pages, and inevitably put it back. Something inside me kept putting it off.

The weekend before radiation was to start, we went to my cousin's wedding in Wisconsin. Her family owned a resort where the wedding and reception were held. It was about five hours away. We arrived late Friday evening after several long hours in the car. I say long hours because we had three kids going stir crazy in the back seat. We only stopped once for gas and supper. Making it five hours in the car is no easy feat with kids. To say the least, we were *all* ready to get out and stretch our legs.

We didn't stay at the resort because it was full with other wedding guests. My cousin had a friend who owned a cabin nearby and she was gracious enough to let us use it for the weekend.

It was down several winding dirt roads. It was pitch black with only the stars and moon offering little light in the dense woods. The cabin was at the end of the dirt road.

We weren't sure if it was the right place. It was in the middle of Nowheresville, Wisconsin, also known as Eagle River. Google Maps showed it was the right place, though; Google knows everything.

I got out and knocked on the door just to make sure we had the right place. Nobody came. I knocked again just to be safe, then slowly cracked the door open.

"Anybody home?" I shouted.

Silence. It was the right place after all. The kitchen light was left on and the door was left unlocked with the keys on the table.

The kids thought it was freaky. I thought it was rustic. I'm sure I would have thought it was scary too if I was their age.

It was late when we arrived. Once we got everything unpacked, we put our pajamas on and went to bed.

The wedding was the next day. We got up early to head to the resort to help out where needed. It looked like it was going to rain. But, the weather gods showed their graces and let the sunshine come out just as the ceremony began.

The reception was in a tented area next to the lodge. The food was excellent and the music was great, too. We spent the night drinking, dancing, and celebrating the nuptials of my cousin and her new husband.

The next morning (Sunday), my parents took Alexis and Tatum home. My wife and I headed to Rochester with the baby. It was another long drive; just over five hours. The baby slept on and off for most of the trip. She started getting fussy towards the end. We stopped a few times to stretch, eat, and let Harper out of her confining car seat.

They stayed with me in a hotel for the first three days. My wife had to get back to St. Cloud for work and she wanted to see the other two girls.

They tagged along for my first three radiation treatments. Kayleigh didn't bring the baby in the waiting area because she didn't want her to spread germs since most of the people in the waiting area had compromised immune systems from radiation and chemo.

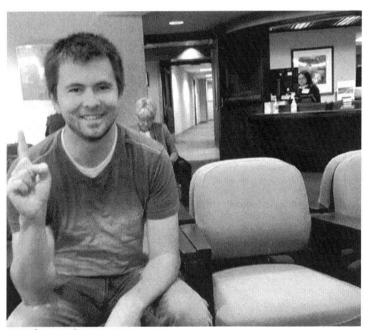

My first radiation treatment.

We hung out for three days and busied ourselves in Rochester. We parted ways on Wednesday after my treatment.

The next six weeks I would be alone. It was a somber ride up the elevator to an empty and eerily quiet room.

Since Rochester was a 2 ½ hour drive from home, we didn't have the money for gas to drive back and forth every day, so I decided to stay down there during the week and come home on the weekends to see my family.

I wasn't allowed to drive for three months after surgery. For some reason, they don't want people who have a high risk of seizures to operate a motor vehicle. Go figure. So, every Monday morning, someone would drive me down and then someone would come back to pick me up on Friday afternoon. Usually, my father-in-law made the trips, but occasionally my dad would take a turn. My aunt, Jeanette, drove me down once as well.

She's a retired oncology nurse. She and I chatted about various types of chemo drugs, because she's familiar with most of them, and their associated side effects. We talked about side effects, different types of cancer, and what drugs were used to treat them and why. She has a wealth of knowledge I eagerly soaked in.

A bridge was being built on Highway 52 on the way to Rochester. I basically got to watch it go up in real time over my treks to and from my treatments for six weeks. Whenever we'd drive down for a follow-up MRI, I always looked at that bridge, now complete, and think about what it looked like when nothing was there. I know, it sounds stupid to reminisce about a bridge, but I did.

Both Doctors, Stafford and Lachance, told us of a place called The Hope Lodge. It's a community for cancer patients who are away from home and need to be in town for treatment. There's no charge to stay there. It was within walking distance of the Mayo Clinic, just two blocks away. We weren't allowed to get on the waiting list until treatment actually started. It used to be that you could get on the list months ahead of time, but they had issues with people abusing it. They changed it so treatment had to actually be underway before you could get on the list.

I lucked out and only had to stay in a hotel for the first week, the week Kayleigh and Harper were with me for the first three days. The next five weeks were at The Hope Lodge.

It was like an apartment building, except there were no kitchens in the units. Just two beds, a small TV with a DVD player (but no cable), a big plush chair, a small table with two chairs, and a bathroom - obviously.

There were four communal kitchens. Every guest was assigned to a kitchen; each kitchen was fully stocked with pots and pans, silverware, cooking utensils, cups, plates, bowls, spices, etc. Anything you'd need to cook a meal was provided. There were about twenty guests per kitchen. Each of us had a shelf in the fridge and the freezer with our room number on it to store food; we were also given a dry storage locker for things that didn't need to be kept cold. There were coffee pots throughout with hot coffee 24-hours a day.

The downstairs of The Hope Lodge had a laundry room for the guests to use, along with a small computer lab to access the Internet. There was Wi-Fi in the building, but I couldn't pick it up in my room. I was forced into the common areas so I could use my iPad to browse Facebook or play games.

The basement also had a huge selection of DVDs and VHS tapes. I hadn't seen a VHS tape in years. I guess they all went to The Hope Lodge in Rochester, because there were hundreds – if not thousands – of them. The movies were free to take up to our rooms to watch and then return to the shelf later. The genre selection was great. I was never without an option for something to watch before hitting the hay. One of the communal televisions was down there as well, along with a pool table, and foosball table.

I realized shortly after I arrived why they didn't have cable TV in the guest rooms. They wanted the guests to mingle and talk, not spend their days wasting away in their rooms watching TV. There were several living areas on the main floor with cable TV hooked up for the guests to share.

The Hope Lodge had a schedule of events each week for the residents to participate in if they wanted. My favorite was the weekly potluck held every Tuesday. I only cooked up a dish for the last one. I felt guilty at first eating everyone's food and not contributing some of my own. That was until I saw how much food a group of cancer patients can produce! There were leftovers for days from each potluck. I didn't feel so bad after all.

I skipped the first potluck because I felt guilty about not having anything to contribute, and I didn't really know anybody yet. I was afraid to sit alone and eat everyone else's food. I started going to them every week after that. I had met some folks by then, and had people to visit with over a hot, home-cooked meal.

I was, by far, the youngest person there. A 30-year-old with brain cancer is not a common thing. I think the next oldest person there was in his mid-40s. I met a lot of great people who could understand what I was going through because they were dealing with the same thing. It was nice being able to speak to people who could truly empathize with what I was going through and what I was feeling, because they were feeling and going through the exact same things.

I had to keep myself to a routine each day to avoid going stir crazy and driving myself insane with loneliness. I didn't set my alarm, but I'd usually wake up around 8 a.m. I'd do some yoga in my room while listening to a local radio morning show. Then I'd shower, shave, get dressed and head down for breakfast. On Wednesdays, I'd call in to the office for our weekly leadership team meeting from 9:00 a.m. to 10:30, then head to breakfast.

There'd be the same folks down there most days. I ate alone for the first week or so. As I warmed up to the other guests, I'd enjoy my breakfast with whoever was down there. We'd share our stories, talk about our families, where we're from, etc. Their stories were varied and unique. There was a couple from China who didn't speak a lick of English. I met a gentleman from Grand Forks, North Dakota where my wife was born. He had throat cancer. Many of the men had prostate cancer. Several women had breast cancer.

I was the only one with brain cancer. Though I was told by another guest that just before I arrived, there was a young lady about my age who also had brain cancer. She checked out the week before I checked in.

Towards the end of my stay, I was in the basement doing some laundry where I met a young woman who was about my age. Early thirties or so, I guessed. She was only staying for a few days with her husband. Her face was sunburnt from whole-head radiation. Whatever cancer she had – I don't remember what it was – ended up moving to her brain. That's why they had to radiate her entire head instead of just a small area.

She had been battling cancer for nearly a decade. She was in her early twenties when she had her first bout with cancer. It kept coming back, so they had to treat it.

"Do you two have any kids?" I asked.

"No," she answered with sadness in her voice. "We've always wanted kids, but that's been on the back burner for a while. Cancer has taken that away from us for now. Hopefully, we'll have kids someday. Just not now. We're trying to stay positive though."

"I'm sorry," I replied. "Kids are a blessing. My wife and I have three daughters. She's at home with them so I can be here."

We talked for a few more minutes before parting ways. After hearing her story, mine didn't sound so bad anymore. It can always be worse. Always.

After breakfast I'd head back up to my room, grab one of the books we'd purchased, and head back down to the library to read a few chapters. I figured if I'm going to be stuck in Rochester, I might as well better myself by reading. Reading is like installing new software in your brain. I was never much of a reader unless I had to for high school or college. I read more books during my stay at The Hope

Lodge than I had the entire previous decade. I've learned to love it and still read on a regular basis now.

Most of the books were about marketing, social media, and leadership and management. I wanted to keep myself sharp for when I returned to work.

I'd read until it was lunchtime, then head over to the kitchen area and make my lunch and chat with the other residents.

My radiation appointments were every day at 1:45. If it was nice out - which it was for the first several weeks - I'd throw my backpack on, and walk over to the building where radiation was. The treatment only took about fifteen minutes. It was weird being down there all week long for just five treatments lasting fifteen minutes each. Each week I had a total treatment time of seventy-five minutes, and yet I was stuck down there, finding ways to kill time for an entire week.

After each treatment was done, I'd put my headphones in and take a long walk while listening to music. I got to know downtown Rochester like the back of my hand. I probably walked over two miles each day. On days when it was cold or raining – or both, I'd walk through the subway systems underneath the Mayo Clinic buildings. By the end of radiation, I had them mapped out perfectly.

That was my routine for the next six weeks. Wake up. Yoga. Shower. Breakfast. Read. Lunch. Treatment. Walk. Dinner. TV. Movie. Bed. Lather, rinse, repeat.

The routine did a great job of keeping the loneliness at bay, except during my first week at The Hope Lodge. I was sitting in the plush chair in the corner of my room, reading a book. I think it was about social media.

I started thinking about how much longer I had to be there, and how much I missed my wife and kids. I put my book down and began to weep. Feelings of loneliness and anguish were rushing through my body. I laid on my bed and cried. It was the first time I had cried since the night we found out about my tumor being a Grade III. All the emotions I had building up while healing at home came rushing out in that moment.

I texted my wife that I had just spent the last half hour crying my eyes out. She called immediately. It was great to hear her voice. We only talked for a few minutes, but it was all I needed to get my head back in the game.

The first several radiation treatments were side-effect free. I'd meet with my radiologist, Dr. Stafford, each Wednesday to discuss how things were going. Most of those meetings were only a few minutes long because I had nothing to report. It got to the point where Dr. Stafford didn't even bother to sit down. I spent more time waiting for him than in the actual appointment.

Eventually, I started losing my taste for certain foods and drinks. Most namely, Caribou Coffee. Which sucked, because I love Caribou, and they had a store across the street from the radiation building.

In the early weeks, I'd head across the street and grab a Caribou before starting my walk, but that stopped when the thought of them started making me nauseated. Other than aversions to certain foods and drinks, I didn't have many other side effects. No headaches (at least not at first), and only minor nausea. It wasn't even severe enough to warrant an anti-nausea pill. Like I said, very minor.

The worst side effect was alopecia. Not sure what that

is? It's the medical term for hair loss. Why they just don't call it hair loss is beyond me. It sure would be easier for the rest of us to understand.

Dr. Stafford told me it would start to happen around week three. Lo and behold, half way through week three, I was in the shower washing my hair and a chunk of it pulled right out. I didn't go totally bald. Alopecia from radiation only effects the area being treated. In my case, I had a bald spot on the front left of my head. That weekend, I had my wife shave my head. It looked much better without thin, patchy spots.

I uploaded before and after pictures to Facebook. Shortly after, Dad texted me a picture. He saw mine on Facebook, and shaved his head in an act of solidarity. My brother soon followed.

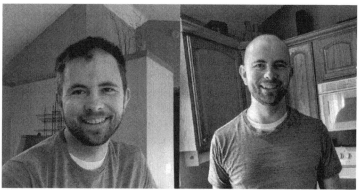

The before and after photos of my haircut. Taken October 5th, 2014.

That Thanksgiving, my hair still hadn't grown back. The doctor thought it could take up to six months. The whole family was gathered at my parent's house. While there, two of my uncles also shaved their heads. We snapped a picture of Dad, my brother, two of my uncles, and me sitting on the floor with our shaved heads. It felt great to have such a strong support system.

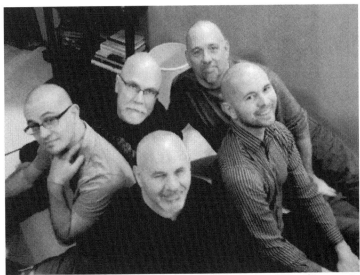

My brother, Aaron on the left. Dad in the middle. Me on the right. Uncle Don top middle, Uncle Pat top right. Heads shaved in solidarity.

Anyway, back to my time in Rochester.

To keep my weeks busy and less mundane, my parents started making weekly trips down to visit every Wednesday. We'd go out to dinner for whatever I was in the mood for because my taste aversions were getting pretty bad. I had cravings for pizza and ice cream mostly. I was like a pregnant woman. I craved only junk food. Why couldn't I crave salad or something healthy for me? I didn't really care that much.

Regardless, I had some company and people I knew coming to visit on a regular basis. It broke up my week and got me out of Downtown Rochester since I couldn't drive anywhere.

Two of my friends came down one Tuesday. I showed them around The Hope Lodge and introduced them to some of the friends I had made. We took in a movie and then went to dinner at a local restaurant and wine bar. Alcohol was the other thing that hadn't been sounding appealing lately. However, I was feeling good that day, so I had a glass of wine with dinner.

We headed back to The Hope Lodge to play some cards. They had to get back to the Twin Cities, about an hour and half north of Rochester, so they left that evening.

An Eventful Day

The next day was a Wednesday. It was October 8th. I remember it well. It started out just like any other day. Same routine. Same everything. My parents were coming down that evening for their weekly visit. They were taking me to dinner. I hadn't decided what I was in the mood for, yet.

After I got back from my daily walk, it was about 3:45 in the afternoon. I headed up to my room to kill time on my laptop until my parents arrived. By this time in my treatment, I was beginning to get headaches from the swelling in my brain. I had one that day, and boy it was a doozy.

To keep my mind away from my headache, and to kill time before my parents arrived, I was playing "Hearthstone" on my laptop. It's a digital card game from Blizzard Entertainment. Yes, I'm that guy. The 30-year-old gamer. Hearthstone kept me occupied when I had nothing else to do and nobody to talk to. I had it on my iPad, as well.

In retrospect, I should have been lying in bed resting my eyes. Screens of any kind – laptops, cell phones, tablets – are not good for headaches. I blame the fact that I wasn't thinking straight. Yeah. That's it.

I remember sitting in my chair at the small table in my room. I was waiting for my opponent to finish his turn. The next thing I knew, I woke up on the floor. I had just passed out.

I laid there for several minutes. Dazed and confused (cue Led Zeppelin). I wondered what the hell had just happened. I felt dizzy and nauseated. I tried to stand up, but couldn't balance myself. I laid there for a few more minutes, then crawled to my bed and struggled to pull myself up.

I was in my bed for a few more minutes. My head was spinning. I was so confused. I couldn't think straight. The first clear thought I had was to call Kayleigh.

"Hi, Babe," I spoke quietly when she answered.

"Honey, what's wrong!?" She could tell by the sound of my voice that something had happened.

"I just passed out."

"You what?!" she asked in shock.

"I just passed out." I said again, still dazed and confused. "I was playing my game...and...and...then I woke up on the floor."

My thoughts and words came slowly. "You were the first person I thought to call."

"Are you okay?" she inquired.

"I think so. I'm shaking and cold."

"Call the clinic. They'll probably have you go in to the E.R. I'll call your parents. I'm sure they're almost there anyway."

After I hung up with my wife, I called the clinic and explained what had just happened. They instructed me to go into the emergency room. When I told them where I was staying, they transferred me down to the front desk at The Hope Lodge.

Once the front desk staff realized I was actually *in* the building, they sent two staffers up to my room. The door was locked, but they had a master key.

By this time, I was able to walk slowly around my room, using furniture to steady myself. I made my way to the bathroom to check the mirror for any bodily damage. I had a nasty scrape on the bridge of my nose and rug burn on the side of my nose. I was bleeding too. I could see where the blood had run down my cheek and dried.

It was odd though. I woke up on my left side, yet the blood had run down the right side of my face. It would have had to go against gravity to do that. I must have lost consciousness, passed out, and had a seizure. That's the only logical explanation for what I saw on my face:

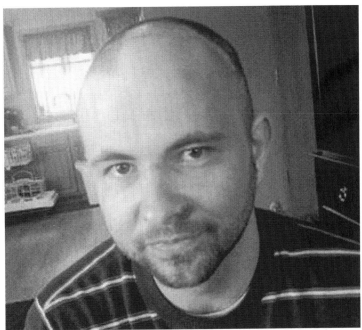

My face after passing out. You can see on the bridge of my nose and the rug burn on the side of my nose. It doesn't look so bad here — but it was awful when it first happened.

I'm not sure how long I was passed out. It must have been a while, because I lost the Hearthstone match due to inactivity and my laptop screen had faded dark, which takes at least ten minutes.

I was in the bathroom when The Hope Lodge staff knocked on the door. It was loud. At least, it sounded loud to me. The headache was probably amplifying any noise entering my ears. I heard the click of the door unlock as they let themselves in.

I made my way out of the bathroom to greet them. I sat on my bed and explained what just happened. I told them my parents were almost here. Kayleigh sent me a text saying they were about fifteen minutes out.

The staffers grabbed a wheelchair for me and took me downstairs to the lobby to wait for my parents.

When my parents arrived, Dad pulled up to the front door while Mom came inside. I told them I had to go into the E.R. Mom wheeled me out to the car and opened the front passenger side door. She helped me in and then took a seat in the back.

The E.R. was in the same hospital where I had my surgery almost exactly two months prior to this. It was about a mile away.

Once the car started moving, I instantly felt nauseated. I asked Mom for something to throw up in. She didn't have anything except a cloth grocery bag. One of the reusable ones. I took it and promptly puked the contents of my stomach into it. I heaved several more times, emptying my belly into the bag. Which then soaked through onto my lap and reeked to high heaven of vomit. Lucky for me, I had my coat on my lap. It took the majority of the leakage instead of my jeans.

Once we arrived at the emergency room, I was put into another wheelchair and given a proper vessel to puke into. A plastic bowl. The E.R. was busy. The line was long. When it was our turn, my mom explained to the folks behind the desk what happened and that I had brain cancer and was staying at The Hope Lodge for radiation treatments. That must have made my case more important than everyone else waiting, because we were taken back to the room right away.

We spent the next several hours in the E.R. getting tests

done. They did an EKG to check my heart, a CT scan to check my head for swelling, and blood work to check for any abnormalities. They all came back normal.

When I was finally discharged, it was well past 10 p.m. and I was starving. Yet again, I was craving pizza. We went to Toppers across the street from the hospital and took it back to The Hope Lodge to eat in the dining area.

I played a game of cribbage with my parents and asked them to stay the night just in case. We watched *The Departed* in my room that night before going to bed.

The next day, we went to visit Dr. Stafford and told him what happened. He believed, based on my description, it was a seizure. He was going to consult with Dr. Lachance though just to be sure. They agreed it was likely a seizure. Since nobody witnessed it and I was passed out for it, there's no way to know for sure. Radiation treatment can cause swelling in the brain, so that explanation makes the most sense.

As a result of their consultations, I was given a prescription for steroids to reduce any swelling the radiation may have caused. They also increased the dose of my anti-seizure pills from 500mg to 750mg.

I'm glad the steroids came when they did, because my headaches were becoming unbearable; to the point where I couldn't think straight because my head hurt so badly from the swelling of my brain. The steroids did their job though. Slowly, the headache intensity faded. Once the tapering dose of steroids was gone, so were the headaches.

Dr. Stafford also told me I can't be alone any more after passing out. I needed to have someone with me at all times in case it happened again.

Mom and Dad stayed that night, too, and drove me home on Friday.

It was nice always having someone there with me. Between my dad, Kayleigh's dad, and my brother, I had someone to stay with me until the end of radiation.

My father joined for one of the potlucks when it was his turn to be my chaperone. He struck up a conversation with one of the other residents. They had nothing in common, but Dad has that unique ability to talk to anyone about anything for as long as they were willing to share. I guess that's why he was in sales for the first part of his career.

MEA Visit

Mid-October is Minnesota Education Association Conference (MEA) for Minnesota schools, which means kids have no school for several days in the middle of the month while teachers attend the conference. Kayleigh used that time to bring the girls down to visit me. They rented a hotel room for a few nights and I got to get out of The Hope Lodge. Not that I didn't enjoy it there, but, obviously, I'd much rather spend time with my family. Plus, kids weren't allowed in The Hope Lodge. It was adults only. They didn't want kids running around, being noisy, and bothering the other guests.

We took the kids back to the area where I was given each radiation treatment and they got to see the mask I wear every day for the ordeal. Tatum thought it was creepy. Alexis thought it was cool. Harper didn't care; she was more interested in either sleeping, or screaming.

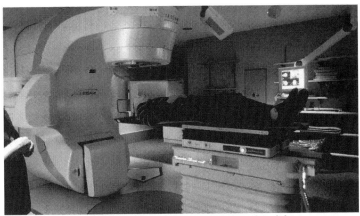

The radiation table. I'd lie here every day for fifteen minutes. The mask on my face was molded to fit my facial features and was fitted with GPS Receivers so the radiation would go exactly where it was meant to. If the beam was off by more than a millimeter, the techs would adjust it. It was a painless procedure. Each treatment had five zones, each requiring the table to rotate and pivot. For one of the zones, I always got a very distinct smell in my nose. It was like bleach or chlorine. It only lasted a few seconds. Very weird.

We also took the girls to a bowling alley and arcade in Rochester. We ordered a couple of pizzas and ate them while we bowled. Just so you know, greasy pizza fingers and bowling don't mix. Slippery fingers lose control of bowling balls. Not that I've ever done that or anything. I'm just saying – you know, for future reference.

I also had my first beer in a long time. A Surly Furious. I didn't finish it. It still didn't taste like I remembered. I avoided alcohol for several weeks after radiation was done.

The next day, we took a trip to Wabasha on the Minnesota border. On the way, we stopped at a unique toy store called Lark Toys. It wasn't like any other toy store I've ever been in. They had a carousel that the kids rode, a gift shop, ice cream parlor, candy store, and various rooms each with different themes for the toys. Many of the toys were made on-site in the wood shop.

The drive was beautiful. Southern Minnesota is a gorgeous site in the fall. We drove through rocky ridges, and followed a road next to a winding river, and we saw eagles soaring in the sky above. Simply breathtaking.

The town of Wabasha (yes, the same Wabasha from the *Grumpy Old Men* movies) was holding their annual fall festival and the bustling town was full of pumpkins and fall colors. There were street vendors, face painting, and a petting zoo.

We visited the National Eagle Center and saw bald eagles up close and personal. The facility was on the banks of the Mississippi River and the area was home to a dense eagle population.

It was great seeing my family for more than a short weekend.

The rest of radiation was uneventful. Since I was required to have someone with me at all times after passing out, someone was always there to keep me company.

The last three days were October 27th–29th of 2014. My wife came down for the last three days. She wanted to be there for my last treatment.

She joined me for the potluck that week. We cooked up a double batch of my famous pesto chicken pasta. It's the only recipe I've created from scratch. I made it once for a contest at work and it won first place. Though, I'll admit, I did tell everyone to vote for my recipe. It's not like I cheated, I just had a better campaign than anyone else.

My favorite part of each potluck was the beginning. Every resident of The Hope Lodge was gathered in the community dining area along with their guests and caretakers. The staff at the lodge would kick things off by asking us to raise our hands if it was our first potluck. Those who raised their hands had the opportunity to introduce themselves, share what kind of cancer they had, and where they were from.

Then, the staff would ask the group to raise their hands if this was their final potluck. Those folks would each take a turn to thank the community and staff for being supportive and endearing for their time at The Hope Lodge.

Most people got choked up as they said their goodbyes and thanked the group. Many of the other residents got teary-eyed as well. I know I did. They had just spent many weeks away from home, going through the worst thing imaginable: cancer. Yet, here in downtown Rochester, was a close-knit community of survivors. People who laid it all out on the line to get better. To heal. They were away from family, and friends. Away from their jobs and hobbies. Away from everything they cared about in life.

I was dreading my last potluck. I knew I'd get emotional. When the staff asked if this was anyone's last potluck, I hesitated. My wife elbowed me in the side, prodding me to raise my hand. So I did. There were a few of us leaving that week. I was the last one to speak.

I don't remember what I said exactly, but I do remember not being able to finish. I immediately choked up and started crying, just like those who spoke before me. I was so thankful for everyone there. The staff, the other residents, The Hope Lodge in general. It was such a blessing - both financially and emotionally - to have that kind of support away from home.

After the potluck, we went back to my room and packed our things. My last treatment was the next day.

There was a bell in the radiation waiting area. Whenever a patient would finish their full treatment schedule, they'd ring the bell, announcing to everyone in the waiting room that treatment was done. Someone rang the bell most days I was down there. The folks waiting in the lobby would cheer as the bell rang. Since everyone in the waiting area was either a family member or a radiation patient themselves, they all knew what it was like. We all shared a commonality. Ringing the bell signified the end of radiation.

Next to the bell was a plaque with the following inscription:

Ring Out

Ring this bell
Three times well
The toll to clearly say
My treatments are done
Its course has run
And I am on my way

On Wednesday, October 29th, I had my final treatment; thirty-three in all. When I walked around the corner into the waiting area, I rang the hell out of that bell! I was looking forward to this moment ever since treatment started six weeks ago. Everyone cheered. I got goosebumps. It felt so good to *finally* be done. The last six weeks were something else. It felt like they dragged on forever, yet, at the same time, they seemed to fly by. It's so strange.

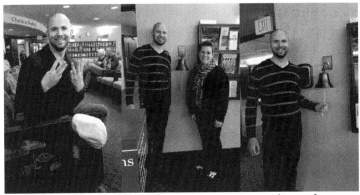

My final radiation treatment. Making a 33 with my fingers to signify 33 treatments completed.

Halloween was that Friday. I returned to work full-time the following Monday. It was great to be back in the saddle, doing what I love with the people I love.

I jumped back into work right where I left off. It felt great to be able to do my job just as I had before, especially after being out for ninety days.

Chemotherapy was scheduled to start in early December, though I'd continue to work full time until April of 2015. Due to the side effects from chemotherapy, I would have to start working from home. Eventually, I'd stop working entirely; no thanks to a particularly nasty side effect called chemo brain.

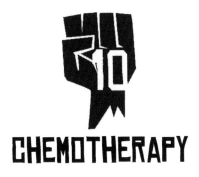

CHEMOTHERAPY

The standard treatment plan for a Grade III Oligoastrocytoma is six weeks of radiation, followed by thirty-six weeks of chemotherapy. Dr. Lachance asked if I'd be willing to participate in a clinical trial for treatment.

The purpose of the trial was to test whether the chemo drug used as standard treatment for Grade IV tumors would work for Grade III tumors. They've had great success treating Grade IV tumors with that particular drug. Their theory was that if it worked so well in Grade IV, it should work the same in Grade III. That drug is called Temozolomide, or Temodar for short. According to my neurologist, it's better tolerated than the chemo cocktail used in Grade III tumors. *Better tolerated.* I liked the sound of that.

The clinical trial consisted of three arms. The first was the standard treatment plan for Grade III tumors. Six weeks of radiation followed by thirty-six weeks of a chemo cocktail called PCV. The second arm was radiation and Temodar together, followed by just Temodar. That was the standard treatment plan for Grade IV tumors. The final arm was just Temodar by itself.

They wanted to test if Temodar had the same positive effects on Grade III tumors, and also test if it had the same effects without subjecting the brain to radiation. If I were to participate in the trial, a computer would randomize me into one of the three trial groups. I would have had a one-in-three chance of taking standard treatment plan for my kind of cancer.

We didn't end up participating because my insurance didn't cover clinical trials. That's something unique to Minnesota. Most other states require insurance companies to cover clinical trials. Not my state. As it turns out, I'm glad we didn't participate in the trial. During one of our subsequent follow-up trips down to the Mayo, Dr. Lachance informed us about a preliminary report he had recently read. The report talked about Grade III tumors treated with Temodar. If they grew back, pathologists would find abnormalities in the genetic makeup of the tumor. Tumors treated with PCV didn't have those if the tumor ended up coming back someday.

Dr. Lachance was elated that we didn't participate in the trial, as were we. Looking back, I knew Someone Upstairs was looking out for us. I'm thankful my insurance didn't cover clinical trials; it made our decision easy. Turns out, it was one of the best decisions we'd ever make.

PCV chemotherapy is a cocktail of three drugs: Procarbazine, Ceenu (aka Lomustine), and Vincristine. Hence PCV. The thirty-six week treatment plan is broken down into six cycles, each six weeks long. Thus, a total of thirty-six weeks. Each cycle is forty-two days.

On Day One, I'd take the Lomustine pills. On days eight and twenty-nine, I had to go into the clinic for an IV infusion of Vincristine. On days eight through twenty-one, I'd take two pills of Procarbazine every day. I'd get a break for the last two weeks and then start the next cycle again on day one.

The dosage of each drug is based on a formula around my height and weight.

Since two of the three drugs were in pill form, I could take them at home. Dr. Lachance referred me to an oncologist at the Coborn Cancer Center in St. Cloud named Dr. Jurgens. Lachance led my treatment remotely from Rochester and Jurgens reported back to him whenever I'd go in for an office visit. It worked out great. I had the expertise of the Mayo Clinic here in my hometown.

One of the drugs, Lomustine, only comes in 10mg, 40mg, and 100mg tablets. My dosage calculated out to 230mg. My doctor in St. Cloud didn't want to give me different pill sizes to avoid any confusion. The only way to get 230mg without mixing pill sizes is to take twenty-three of the 10mg pills. So, that's what I did. I took twenty-three pills on day one of each chemo cycle. I'm pretty sure I could figure out two 100mg and three 10mg pills. Oh well. It was only on the first day of each cycle.

During the first cycle, Dr. Jurgens asked me to come in each week for a blood draw. He wanted to see how the chemo drugs were effecting my blood counts. One of the many doctors I saw down at the Mayo told me, "PCV Chemotherapy is like a sledgehammer to the immune system." I could see why Dr. Jurgens wanted a blood test every week.

I was also given a prescription for anti-nausea pills. I was instructed to take one about an hour before I took my chemo pills and then every six to eight hours thereafter, as needed for nausea.

Lomustine

On Friday, December 5th, I popped an anti-nausea pill. Then, an hour later, twenty-three pills of Lomustine went down the hatch; kicking off cycle one.

To my surprise, I didn't feel nauseated much at all. Each cycle started on a Friday so I could have the weekend to be sick if need be. I had it scheduled like that intentionally. Lomustine is the drug which tends to cause nausea in most patients. Followed by Procarbazine. Vincristine, the IV-injected drug, didn't have nausea as a common side effect.

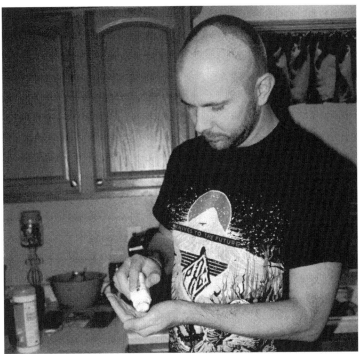

December 5th, 2014. Day One, Cycle One of chemo. Twenty-three Pills of Lomustine. You can clearly see my surgery scar and the area where I was treated for radiation.

The next day, I took my daughter to a hockey tournament in Paynesville; about a 45-minute drive from our house. I wasn't able to drive yet, so my dad and brother tagged along with Tatum and me. I downed an anti-nausea pill just in case when we left on Saturday morning.

My stomach was a little irritated, but nothing even remotely close to making me vomit. Honestly, I was surprised. I've heard horror stories of chemo patients spending several agonizing nights over the toilet, puking their guts out. I was expecting to have the same experience. I didn't.

I went into work on Monday morning with an anti-nausea pill at the ready, but never ended up needing it. It sat on my desk for months. The pills work quickly. The instructions on the bottle were to take one when nausea starts. I never once felt nauseated that first week after chemo started. I was getting excited that I may not be one of the horror stories.

On Friday, December 12th, I went into the Coborn Cancer Center for a blood draw, office visit, and the first infusion of Vincristine. Dr. Jurgens reviewed my lab results with Kayleigh and me. My blood counts had actually gone up!

"If this trend continues," Dr. Jurgens explained, "you'll have an easy six cycles of chemo."

I hoped he was right.

It later turned out that he was wrong. Very wrong.

Vincristine

After the office visit, I headed back to the lobby to wait for my infusion. My wife and I went to the clinic on days eight and twenty-nine of every cycle and spent most of the morning waiting. Each visit would last no less than two hours. I learned to bring a book with after the first two visits.

The first Vincristine infusion was awful. The clinic has a chemotherapy infusion area with about forty rooms, each equipped with a comfortable chair and a television. Most chemo patients are at the infusion lab for hours on end because their drugs take that long to infuse. My infusion only took five minutes. The wait was longer than the actual infusion.

I was nervous the first time. Aren't we all nervous the first time? I've had IV's before, but none like this. Plus, I was there in the morning, so I hadn't had anything to drink since the night before. I was dehydrated and my veins were hard to stick.

They couldn't use the vein in the crook of my arm because Vincristine is a caustic drug. If it gets out of the vein and into the surrounding tissue, it'll start to break it down and cause chemical burns right in front of your eyes. I imagine it hurts like hell too. The crook of the arm, while a huge vein, wasn't a safe place to insert the IV. I didn't want them to use the veins in my wrist. I was too scared. I asked about the veins in my forearm. Those would be fine. They put a hot pack onto my arm to loosen up the veins and bring them to the surface. The nurse wrapped a tourniquet around my elbow to make the veins stick up even more, just like they do when drawing blood. Only this time, their target was much smaller.

The first nurse who stuck me hit a valve in my vein. She pushed the needle in. Pulled it back. Pushed. Pulled. Twisted. It stung every time she moved the needle. She couldn't get it into the vein. She tried my other arm and another hot pack.

I was shaking and cold, which only made it worse. She couldn't find any veins. My veins must have a mind of their own, because they disappeared whenever I sat down in the infusion chair, even if I was fully-hydrated and not a jittery, nervous mess. I've been told many times that I have great veins, so I'm not really sure what was going on when I went in for Vincristine.

Each nurse was only allowed two attempts to get an IV in. Once their two tries were over, they needed to call another nurse in. The nurse she called over got the IV in right away. No pain or pinching. I liked her. Too bad I couldn't choose the nurse every time.

Once the IV was in, they started a saline drip to keep the vein from closing up while we waited for the pharmacy to send the Vincristine bag up. Being there so early every morning meant we didn't need to wait long for the pharmacy to get the drug mixed and bagged for us.

I was surprised at how small the Vincristine bag was. My dosage was only 50 milliliters. Typically, they give it along with other chemo infusions. For me, I only had to get the Vincristine. It only takes five minutes for 50ml to run, plus another five minutes for a saline flush. Ten minutes and I was done. Like I said, we spent more time waiting than we did getting the actual infusion.

The rest of my infusions weren't nearly as bad as the first one. There were a couple when the nurse didn't get the IV to stick the first try, but she got it the second time. Most of the time, though, the IV's went in just fine right away.

The biggest side effects from Vincristine are hair loss, neuropathy of the extremities, and constipation. Neuropathy is another one of those medical terms I learned. It is numbness and loss of feeling in certain parts of the body. The constipation comes from neuropathy of the gut. Dr. Jurgens and Dr. Lachance both told me that neuropathy can be permanent in many cases. If it ever got to a point where I couldn't function or walk because of it, they'd just stop the Vincristine and continue with the other two drugs.

Vincristine was, according to my doctors, the drug with the least effect on treating brain cancer. The only reason I needed to take it was because it was used in the study that made PCV the standard treatment for Grade III brain tumors.

As for hair loss, I was also expecting to go completely bald. Like, queue-ball bald, smooth and shiny. It never happened. I guess the dosage was just too small to make my hair fall out. I'd have to live with a bald spot from radiation, and shortly buzzed hair on the rest of my head until my bald spot started to grow back. It took a few months, but it all came back.

I was told that hair loss from radiation will likely grow back differently than it was before. It could come back thicker or thinner, grow in a different direction, or even be a different color. I lucked out for the most part. Mine grew back thinner and softer than before, and in a slightly different direction. Thankfully, it didn't change color. It would have been awkward having a patch of blonde hair, or worse, a patch of gray. I've already got too many of those.

Procarbazine

Also that day, after work, I started fourteen days' worth of Procarbazine. I took two pills, each 50mg every day for two weeks. With that drug, I also took anti-nausea pills. If you're not familiar with anti-nausea drugs, they don't have many side effects. I was prescribed two types of drugs and was instructed to alternate between them as needed for nausea.

The listed side effect for one of the drugs was dizziness. The other one caused constipation. That's the one I took for the Lomustine because it lasted for eight hours and my doctor told me to start with that one. So I took it every day for the Procarbazine too. Big mistake.

I was blocked up like a brick wall for days. I ended up buying stool softeners, but misread the dosage instructions. I know what you're thinking: I took too many and lived out the scene from *Dumb & Dumber* when Harry had a massive diarrhea explosion in Mary's bathroom, complete with sound effects, gurgles, and screams, finally culminating in a plugged up toilet and a massive stench that could kill a horse.

No. Not quite. I misread the directions the other way. I took the dose for children, one pill. I was still backed up. So backed up that it hurt up into my gut.

After four days, the pain was agonizing. That's when I decided to re-read the dosage instructions on the stool softeners. The adult dose was two to four pills! I promptly downed four pills with a big cup of water.

An hour later, they kicked in. When stool softeners kick in, they don't give a warning. Nothing. Not even a, "Hey, we're about to vacate your bowels, better get to the bathroom." They just go, and if you're not close to a toilet, you'd better have a change of clothes. Luckily, I was close to a toilet.

I won't get into the details of my bowel activities any further than I already have. I did feel great afterwards, though.

Once I got the hang of using the stool softeners in conjunction with the anti-nausea pills, the rest of the first cycle of Procarbazine was smooth sailing.

There was one thing I noticed: I didn't feel nauseated at all. Perhaps Procarbazine just didn't make me feel sick?

Cycle Two

On January 16th, 2015, I started cycle two with twenty-three more pills of Lomustine. I took an anti-nausea pill that time, too. I still didn't feel very nauseated. I began to think I might just be in the clear for chemo's nasty side effects.

The following Friday, the Vincristine infusion went much better than the first one. One poke, no pain. In and out in thirty minutes. Again, most of that time was spent waiting for the pharmacy to mix the drug and send it up to the infusion area.

I was also to start fourteen days' worth of Procarbazine that evening. Remembering the awful constipation experience from cycle one, I took a gamble. I didn't take any anti-nausea pills. The gamble paid off. Turns out, Procarbazine just didn't make me feel sick. I felt great. I was kicking cancer's ass left and right. Nothing could bring me down.

My blood counts didn't change much after cycle one. They went down a little bit, but were still well within the normal range. The anti-nausea pills worked for the Lomustine – though I still had a sneaking suspicion that chemo drugs in general just don't make me sick. I had a great infusion. I didn't need anti-nausea pills for the Procarbazine. Perhaps having cancer at such a young age has some benefits after all!

My nurse at the clinic told me that age is definitely a factor. So is alcohol consumption. People who drank more tended to get sick less while on chemo. I guess their stomachs were already accustomed to feeling nauseated and had adapted to the feeling. I didn't drink like a fish or anything like that, but as an avid homebrewer and self-proclaimed craft beer aficionado, I enjoyed a tasty beer or two on a regular basis.

Much to my chagrin, I wasn't supposed to drink anything while on Lomustine or Procarbazine. I did, however, have a two-week period at the end of each cycle where I was able to drink. I took full advantage of that period in the first two cycles. Once the rest of the cycles came around, I lost all taste for beer – and for food in general. I began losing weight.

Everything I've read about eating while on chemo says to have several small meals throughout the day instead of three larger ones. I tried to stick to that plan the best I could. I'd have a protein shake – Shakeology from Beachbody – and a banana for breakfast. I figured the high density of nutrients in Shakeology plus the banana would give me energy for the day. Then I'd have a mid-morning snack, a light lunch, an afternoon snack, and then a full meal for supper. As much as I tried to eat smaller meals more often, it just didn't help. I simply wasn't hungry.

When I started chemo, I weighed 185 pounds. When I finished chemo, the scale read 160 pounds. I dipped down into the upper 150s for a week or so in there towards the end, too.

I've always had a goal of getting my weight down to 175 and to tone up a little bit. If you're looking for a way to lose weight quickly, I highly recommend the chemo diet! I lost twenty-five pounds in five months! Whenever I look in the mirror, I can see my ab. Yes, I said ab. Singular. One. I can also see my rib cage. Not so cool. Oh well, 160 is still a healthy weight for someone my size – albeit on the low end of healthy.

I also did yoga most mornings to keep myself active. Nothing too strenuous like weightlifting or cardio; I didn't want to lose even more fat. I needed to keep it on, yet stay active at the same time. Yoga was a perfect exercise to do just that.

After cycle two, my blood counts dropped. They bounced up quickly in the two week period I had between cycles, but not quite as high as they were before. They came up enough so I can start the next chemotherapy cycle.

But, I could see the beginning of a trend. A trend that would wind me up in the emergency room.

Cycle Three

This cycle started - as usual - on a Friday. February 27th, to be exact. Same routine as before. I still felt good, my blood counts were decent. I continued working full time, hoping that the blood count trend wouldn't get much worse.

The trend we saw was that my counts dipped further and further after each cycle, and came back up less and less before the next cycle. Each cycle had a minimum level for each particular blood count. White blood cells, red blood cells, platelets, hemoglobin, absolute neutrophil count, etc. Each had a minimum range that needed to be met before I could proceed with treatment.

All of my counts were just within the minimum range when I started cycle three, but not by much.

I had a few more blood draws during this cycle just to monitor my counts throughout treatment. My platelets and white blood cell counts dropped to dangerously low levels when I had a blood draw on day twenty-nine before I went in for the second Vincristine infusion of the cycle. They had a couple weeks to bounce back up.

I must have been lucky, because people with low white blood cells counts are more susceptible to getting sick. We had some bug that ran through our entire house – everyone was sick except for me. In fact, I avoided any sort of sickness for the entire time I was going through cancer treatment. Not your average cancer patient experience.

Low platelet counts also cause people to bruise much easier and to bleed continuously when cut. With as low as mine were, I should have bruised whenever I touched something with any amount of force, but that never happened. Fortunately, I've never bruised very easily my entire life. Now wasn't any different.

I did bleed more after my blood draws – a couple times I bled through the bandaged gauze. Still, nothing major.

At the end of this cycle, a week after my last infusion, I went to a quarterly management team meeting at my boss's house. It was an all-day affair. I was doing great during the morning. I was alert, asking questions, and actively involved in the discussions.

When we took a break for lunch, I could feel myself getting tired. I had worked my brain all morning long and my body felt it. I had a headache, and couldn't think clearly. I was groggy, my eyes glazed over. I didn't say much the rest of the day. I tried hard to pay attention, but was having a difficult time concentrating. I don't even remember the last part of the day.

We walked across the street to a local brewery afterwards to celebrate a long day of hard work and good discussions. I ordered a beer, but struggled to finish it. I sat quietly. I only spoke when spoken to. My answers were short; I was visibly tired. My boss even remarked that I looked tired. I nodded with a yawn.

I crashed on the couch when I got home that evening. It was becoming a common occurrence for me.

Chemo Brain

In mid-March, my boss asked me to start working reduced hours from home. We decided to wait until early April before the reduced hours began to give the rest of the company time to prepare for my new schedule. I only came into the office on Wednesdays for our leadership team meetings, and on Fridays for our client Beerstorming sessions – though I didn't drink beer because the thought of it made me feel sick.

He kept noticing things that I didn't – or perhaps that I refused to see. It got to the point where he just couldn't have me working at the office full time. It wasn't safe for me to keep pushing myself.

"You need to take care of yourself," he told me. "You're in the fight of your life! You should be at home resting."

He was right – but I refused to believe that anything was wrong. I didn't feel sick. I didn't look sick. I wasn't laid up in bed, puking my guts out. I *felt* fine. That was the lie I kept telling myself.

I was so hell bent to go through all of chemo without any side effects that I was blinded by it. Others around me could clearly see that I was struggling cognitively and emotionally. My wife could see it. My boss could see it. My colleagues could see it. I refused to see it. I didn't want to see it.

Chemo brain is a well-documented condition, though it has only recently been studied by oncologists and scientists. There's no doubt it exists. Up to 80% of cancer patients report it as a side effect of chemotherapy.

The best way to describe it is a mental fog. You can't think straight. You're confused. You take longer to form a thought and then express that thought with words. You get tired easily. You struggle to find the right words, etc.

Many of those side effects are also part of having low blood counts. I took a lot of naps during chemo.

Chemo brain itself is irritating to deal with. But for me, since I also have brain cancer, the side effects from the surgery and radiation to my head played into the intensity of chemo brain. It's a double dose of suck.

Oh, you're having side effects from having your brain cut open? Here's chemo brain, too! Thanks, Cancer. I hate you even more now.

In retrospect, I could feel the effects of chemo brain back in cycle two. They were probably there in cycle one, but not strong enough for anyone to notice. The side effects only got worse from then on.

They were easy to hide at first. Eventually, as I got more and more tired, and as my blood counts dropped - as chemo brain became worse, it was impossible to hide. I was embarrassed. I wasn't able to do the things I used to do. I wasn't able to think or solve problems like I used to do. I didn't want my coworkers or family to know. Being physically sick is one thing. People understand that – they can *see* it. If they can see it, they can empathize with it. Being mentally and emotionally sick – that's an entirely different ball game.

I used to be sharp and focused. I could get in the zone and work on something for hours on end. Then I could report back about what I did, and explain it in terms non-technical folks could easily understand. I was no longer capable of that level of mental exertion, or that level of clearly and simply articulating complex topics. It was one of the things I was best at, and I feared it would never come back.

I'd like to say that chemo brain goes away once chemotherapy is over. It doesn't. Some people report mental fogginess issues for years after treatment is done. For others, they're back to normal within a few months. For me, it's getting better every day. I'm optimistic about the long term outlook of my chemo brain.

Cycle Four

This cycle started on Friday, April 10th. I was working reduced hours from home at this time, as well.

My blood counts barely came back within range for this cycle. They were scarcely on the low end of the range. Throughout cycles three and four, I was noticeably more tired. When I'd get home from work, I'd lie on the couch and fall asleep. I lost all interest in playing with my kids, talking to my wife, working out in the morning, and helping out around the house.

I just wanted to lie around and do nothing. Rest my eyes. Watch Netflix. Be lazy. Take the easy road.

I had cancer, after all. I could be selfish for a while. That's what I kept telling myself to justify not wanting to do anything. I was starting to get depressed.

Cycle Five was supposed to start on May 22nd. I went in

for a blood draw to verify that my blood counts had come back up. They hadn't. They were all well below the normal range. In fact, my platelet count dropped to twenty-four. The normal range is at least 150. All of my levels were dangerously low. No wonder I was so sluggish and tired.

I couldn't start the next cycle with my blood counts that low. Dr. Jurgens had me wait a week and then we'd test them again. So, on Friday, May 29th, I went in for another blood draw. My levels were still dropping. All of them were down even further. My platelets were at eighteen. My doctor didn't think they'd come back within range by the next week.

"Let's wait until June 15th," he suggested. "I highly doubt your counts will increase as much as we need them to over the next week. Let's give it a couple weeks and we'll check again. I'm on vacation the second week of June. Can you come back on Monday the 15th for another blood draw?"

"That works," I begrudgingly replied. I was already pissed that treatment had been delayed by a week. Now it was delayed by two more weeks. I only had two cycles left and I wanted them to be over with. I had to wait even longer to find out if we could start the next cycle.

Are we going to go through this again at the end of cycle five? I thought to myself.

Dr. Jurgens interrupted my thoughts. "I'd also like to give you a shot to help boost your white blood cell production. We can do that today before you leave."

That shot was called GRANIX. It is given to patients with neutropenia, a condition where neutrophils are low and need to be boosted. Neutrophils are the most abundant part of the white blood cell, and they're a critical component to the immune system.

Cancer patients are among the most common candidates for GRANIX for obvious reasons. It works in the larger bones of the body to stimulate white blood cell production.

They did the injection back in the chemo infusion area. The nurse had to inject it gradually. A quick injection would burn like hell. It took a good five minutes for her to finish the shot into the triceps on my left arm. I could feel it starting to burn towards the end. It was more of a pinch than a burn. It began to escalate with intensity as the shot progressed.

I winced in pain and shrunk down in my chair, trying not to move my left arm. My wife apologized for laughing at me. The look on my face must have been hilarious. It was finally over and the nurse pulled the needle from my burning arm. The pain went away instantly.

"You might feel some bone pain as this kicks in later tonight," she explained, "mainly in your sternum and femur bones, since those are among the largest in the body."

I didn't feel much of anything until we went to bed that night. Then it felt like someone was sitting on my chest. It was hard to breathe, and hurt if I took big breaths. I laid on my back and tried to breathe slowly. I was already tired from my day, so I fell asleep quickly, despite the pain.

Tuesday, June 2nd

My sister-in-law, Sophia, was our nanny for the summer. She came over at 7:30 each morning and I would retreat to the downstairs office to get a few hours of work in for the day. I'd have a protein shake and a banana for breakfast because my appetite wasn't what it used to be. I had to eat smaller meals more often. That was the weekly routine when summer vacation started.

This day followed that same routine. When Sophia arrived, I went down to the office for a yoga workout. I don't remember if I actually did it or not, though. I wasn't in the mood to do much of anything. I had to force myself to keep both my body and my mind busy. I probably just farted around on my computer for a while. I went back upstairs to make my shake and eat a banana. I took the shake down to the office to finish it while I got some work done.

About mid-morning, I began feeling nauseated, which was odd because I hadn't taken any chemo drugs for almost a month. I've learned that when it comes to chemotherapy, nothing is surprising.

I closed my eyes and began to breathe through my nose, trying to calm my nausea. It subsided slightly. I took that window of opportunity to head upstairs and grab a Tupperware bowl just in case I needed something to spew into.

Back downstairs, I started working again – only for the nausea to return. I closed my eyes again, and breathed through my nose slowly. It wasn't working. I got into the fetal position on the floor, bowl at the ready, eyes still closed. I started to feel pain in my abdomen.

I couldn't control my nausea any longer. I threw up into

the Tupperware bowl. The heaving made my abdomen ache even more. I threw up again. I laid on my office floor in agony. No position was comfortable.

I forced myself to stand and make my way upstairs – trying to avoid my kids since I'm sure I looked miserable. I headed back to our bedroom and closed the door, then collapsed on my bed. I was freezing, so I shivered my way under the blankets. The pain in my abdomen was getting stronger. I tossed and turned, trying to get comfortable.

I sat up, and instantly the nausea came back. I fell onto the floor and puked again into the Tupperware container. I made my way into the bathroom to dump the container into the toilet. I managed to do so, but then puked again - into the toilet this time. I flushed, then rinsed out the container in the sink. I laid on the bathroom floor for a while, trying to get comfortable.

Eventually, I crawled back out onto my bedroom floor. The pain in my abdomen was agonizing. The pain had spread all over - my sides, my stomach, my back. It was concentrated directly behind my belly button, and radiated from there. I was still shivering. I reached up and dragged the blanket off the bed. I slowly draped it over my aching body, trying to find a comfortable position.

Nothing worked.

The pain just kept getting worse. I texted Kayleigh and explained what was going on.

Call the clinic, she responded. Duh.

I called and asked for Dr. Jurgen's nurse. I told them it was urgent. The clinic patched me through to the on-call nurse for the cancer center. I explained to her what was going on.

"Can you describe the level of pain you're in right now?" she asked.

"On a sale of 1 to 10," I groaned, "it's a 12."

I had never been in so much pain in my life. Agonizing doesn't even begin to describe it. It was the worst thing I've ever experienced, and it was throughout my entire lower abdomen and back.

"Head to the emergency room," she instructed.

After I hung up, I texted my wife back.

They want me to go to the E.R.

She replied almost immediately. She was going to leave work right away to come get me. She actually worked at the hospital, so she had to leave and then go right back with me. I was in no condition to drive.

I had been able to drive since January 8th, three months after passing out in my room at The Hope Lodge. That's what the law requires. No driving for three months after an "unexplained loss of consciousness."

I continued to lie on the floor for several minutes, trying to find a way to make the pain in my gut go away.

Then, things took a turn for the worse. I had to shit. Now.

I scrambled to the toilet and sat down. My bowels vacated promptly. It was all liquid. I had the Hershey Squirts. Diarrhea.

Great, I thought, *now it's coming out of both ends!*

I sat on the toilet until Kayleigh arrived. I kept breathing through my nose in an attempt to keep the nausea at bay. I rocked back and forth, trying to offer some comfort to my abdomen.

We had to wait until I felt like I was ready to leave. No

nausea, nothing in my gut telling me to sit on the toilet. I was still shivering cold.

Finally, I was able to settle enough to put some clothes on so we could head to the hospital. I was in sheer agony the entire drive. I took another bowl with just in case. I closed my eyes the whole drive to keep my queasy stomach from churning in the moving car. Two trips to the emergency room in less than a year. Lucky me.

By the time we arrived, I could barely move. My gut was in so much pain, and I was afraid to fart because of the diarrhea.

There was a metal detector and security guard at the entrance to the E.R. I'm glad there wasn't a line. You'd think they would let someone right through in an emergency, but no. I had to take out my keys, and remove my belt and wallet before limping painfully through the metal detector. The guard had Kayleigh do the same after checking her purse.

By this time, the pain in my abdomen had gone from a constant, excruciating pain, to a come-and-go, excruciating pain. As we sat in the admitting room, my wife had to answer for me if my gut pain started to come back. I couldn't think straight with that much pain. Kayleigh explained to the admitting nurse everything I was experiencing, and that I was currently taking chemotherapy for brain cancer.

I was in a wheel chair at this point because I could hardly walk without stopping and doubling over every few steps from the pain. They led us back to one of the rooms and had me put on a hospital gown, then stuck me with an IV for fluids; standard fare in the emergency room.

Shortly after we were in the room, between my fits of pain and nausea, Kayleigh told me we should probably tell my parents what's going on. I'm sure they'd want to know if their son with cancer was in the emergency room.

They had texted us the night before saying they were in a hospital in the Twin Cities with Uncle Greg and his wife, Candy. He was having complications from his cancer. A few other family members were also there. This would likely be the day he passed away.

Now what do we do? My parents are supporting a close family member on his cancer death bed. And here I was, in the emergency room on the same day because of cancer. We can't tell them I'm here. We have to tell them I'm here. They'd be crushed if they later found out I was in the E.R. and we didn't let them know.

We decided to tell them. If things took a turn for the worse, they would want to be here with me.

Kayleigh texted Dad. He's the logical one between my parents. He'd let Mom know for us. While it wouldn't stop either of them from getting emotional, or from thinking the worst, it was the best course of action in that moment.

This is what she sent to him:

Hey guys. I saw that you're in the hospital with Greg and Candy. We're sorry to hear that! Give Candy a hug for us. I hate to burden you with more bad news, but Trav is in the E.R. right now. He was puking uncontrollably and having major abdominal pain. They sent us here just to be safe. We'll keep you posted.

One of the doctors came in to examine me and ask some questions. By this time, the pain in my abdomen would come and go. I was able to sit for a few minutes and feel totally fine, then the pain would gradually increase. I'd have to squirm around the small bed, trying to ease the pain the best that I could.

"Given your history," the doctor started, "I'd like to run some tests to rule out some things. I'd like you to get an ultrasound to look for gall stones, and an abdominal CAT scan to see if there's anything going on in there that we might need to have surgery for."

Fantastic, I thought sarcastically, *more surgery!*

"What have you had to eat today?" he asked.

"Just a banana and a protein shake," I replied. It was well past lunchtime at this point, but I wasn't the least bit hungry.

"Have you had those before?" the doctor went on.

"Lots of times."

"Hmm. Well I doubt it's food poisoning if you've had them before. Let's run those tests just to be sure."

The pain in my abdomen was beginning to get weaker. We had been at the E.R. for two hours already before the first test was performed.

I had the ultrasound first. By then, my abdominal pain was essentially gone. But, my stomach would gurgle and I'd have the urge to pass gas every few moments. I was afraid of what would happen if I did.

The ultrasound tech had me lean to my left side so she could examine the part of my abdomen where my gall bladder sits. It was neat seeing my insides on the screen. The only times I ever saw ultrasounds were when my wife had them for our children. I've never actually seen my own insides before. Come to think of it, I've had brain surgery. It's *my* brain and I never got to see it!

The tech had to push and prod. Her pushing on my gut made the urge to fart even stronger. I held it back as long as possible. My belly gurgled as whatever was inside moved into my intestines. I squirmed as she applied more pressure with the ultrasound wand.

I couldn't hold it anymore. I tried to pass gas quietly, but it wasn't just gas. I sharted.

Dammit! I thought, *I bet this is going to be a long day. I'm sure that won't be the only time I do that.*

When the ultrasound was over, I was taken to the CAT scan area. The two techs in here, again both girls, instructed me to lie on the table and put my arms over my head.

Why did both tests have to be done by all girls? It was bad enough that I had it coming out of both ends, but in front of girls too? That's just mean.

They attached something to my IV that would be injected mid-scan.

"Have you ever had X-Ray dye before?" one of them asked.

"Never even heard of it."

"Well, you'll feel it going in, but, just as a warning, it'll make you feel like you're peeing your pants. Don't worry, you really aren't!"

"Looking forward to it," I joked.

Once my arms were over my head and the X-Ray dye attached to my IV, both techs retreated to the control room. The scan only lasted a few minutes. There were instructions on the machine telling me to hold my breath for a few seconds and then exhale slowly. I did that a few times before the dye was injected.

They weren't kidding. I felt like I was pissing my pants. It's amazing how your mind can be tricked so easily into feeling something that's not really happening.

The scan was over shortly thereafter.

"That's a very odd sensation!" I told the techs. They both laughed. I'm sure they hear it all the time.

Back in my room, my stomach was doing somersaults. The abdominal pain was gone by this point. Now, the diarrhea took over. My belly kept gurgling and settling, the urge to fart was constant. I tried to let a few out, but they were all squishy. Yep. Embarrassing. A grown man soiling his pants. I felt gross.

I told my wife. She laughed a little, but quickly apologized.

"I'm going to need a change of clothes," I told her.

"I'll text my parents and have them bring some over."

"Really? You're going to tell your parents that I shit my pants?"

"Do you have another option?"

"No...I guess not," I replied, embarrassment in my voice.

"Do you need to use the bathroom?" she asked.

"I'm afraid to move. I don't want to disturb whatever the hell is going on down there."

A doctor interrupted our conversation about bodily functions.

"Both tests came back normal. No gall stones, nothing abnormal in the CAT scan," he informed us. "How do you feel now?"

"Like I need to sit on the toilet. I have messy farts."

"Sounds like it's moving through your system," the doctor replied. "I'd like to get a stool sample."

"Alright. I'll let you know when I need to go."

Long story short, I made it to the bathroom, gave them a stool sample, and changed into the new clothes Kayleigh's parents dropped off for me.

We were discharged well after dinner time, but I still wasn't hungry.

As we packed our things, Kayleigh got a text message from my parents.

Uncle Greg had just passed away.

June 3ʳᵈ

The next morning, I felt great. It was as if nothing had ever happened, like I had never been to the emergency room. Cancer. Go figure.

Since I felt fine, I went into the office for our weekly leadership team meeting. I had been working part-time from home during all of this.

During that meeting, the leadership team had a Come to Jesus talk with me. They all agreed I should stop coming in to the office on Wednesdays and Fridays and stop working entirely until treatment was done. It was beyond the point of no return. I was providing zero value by being there. My work at home was suffering too. Chemo brain was at its worst. Nobody had the heart to bring it up sooner. I wish they would have.

They wanted me to put myself first, put my family first. They knew I needed to focus on getting better - on kicking cancer's ass. I didn't like any of it, but I didn't have a choice in the matter either. Deep down, I knew they were right. I just refused to see it and to grasp the reality of my situation. I was living in a bubble. A happy, cancer-free bubble with butterflies, pink roses, and lollipops.

After that meeting, I stopped working entirely. No meetings, no email, no phone calls. Nothing. I tried to focus on my health and getting better, but I only got more depressed. I wanted to be at work so bad that it brought me to tears many times.

Being at work made me feel normal. It made my life feel less chaotic, less of a mess. It wasn't doing me any good, though. I was only hurting myself by showing up twice a week.

The next week, on June 10th, my boss - along with the president of Leighton Enterprises and our human resources guru - presented me with the return to work plan they had been working on for me. It was broken down into four phases, each thirteen weeks long.

When treatment was over - when I felt ready - I could begin working from home again on internal tasks. When I was ready to begin Phase 1, with approval from my doctor, I would start working one day per week in the office.

Phase 2 was two days per week in the office.

Phase 3 was three days per week in the office.

Phase 4 was full-time.

After each phase, I'd have a review to look at my progress and to assess, again with permission from my doctor, if I was ready to move to the next phase in the plan.

I hated it. I hated that it was so long. I hated that I didn't have a say in it. I hated all of it.

It would be a full year before the entire plan was over. Each phase was twice as long as each chemo cycle. It was too damn long! I was sick and tired of having cancer, of going through radiation, and of being sick from chemo. I wanted all of it to be over and done with. I wanted to be back at work – full-time – more than anything in the world. This plan would drag that out more than a year.

When I got home, I promptly Googled information on how long it takes to recover from chemotherapy, and how long the effects of chemo brain can last. I was determined to find something I could use as ammo against the plan.

I didn't like what I found. I discovered why the plan was laid out the way it was. While I didn't find any statistics about cancer recovery time, I did find a forum about cancer recovery. There were hundreds of posts. Some reported being back to normal a few months after treatment was over. For others, it took years before they felt like they were back to their old self again. By and large, the average recovery time was about a year. That's why the plan was phased out over a year. I started to understand.

I still didn't like it, but at least I understood.

Then, I emailed the three guys I met with, thanked them for their time, and asked a few follow-up questions about the plan.

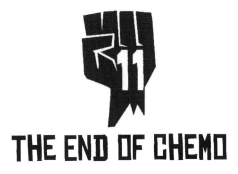

THE END OF CHEMO

I had been waiting for June 15th for over two weeks. It was the day I'd find out if I could start Cycle 5. The last couple of weeks had gone by so slowly. Time seemed to drag on and on.

I went to the clinic that afternoon for a blood draw, and then met with Dr. Jurgens at 2:30 to review the results.

All of my levels were back within normal range except for two, but both were related. My white blood cell count was still dangerously low, as was my absolute neutrophil count (ANC). Dr. Jurgens gives more weight to the ANC than to any other count. Those are my "fighter cells" he called them.

A normal range for those is anything above 1.2. At 0.7, mine were in the danger zone. If they got down to 0.5 or lower, my life could be in serious jeopardy. He didn't want to start the next cycle until both counts came back up.

Then, we talked about my platelets. They bounced back up to 145. Slightly lower than normal, but still pretty good for a guy with cancer. They had dropped down to eighteen before. Dr. Jurgens feared they would drop even further during cycles five and six; which brought up a new concern: once platelets drop into the single digits, a very real possibility, I run the risk of sudden bleeding in the brain. This can cause, among other not so nice things, death.

"We can't continue treatment until the white blood cells and ANC's are back up. When we do, it'll be a half dose of each drug. That said, have you put any thought into stopping treatment?" he asked.

I looked at Kayleigh, then back at Dr. Jurgens. "Not really," I replied. "I'm open to it if that's what you and Dr. Lachance recommend. We came in here expecting to either be delayed again, or to be given the go-ahead to start the next cycle. The thought of stopping never even occurred to us."

"I'll email Dr. Lachance to get his opinion. What I can tell you, though, is that even if you decide to continue, it'll be a half dose of each drug. Even with a half dose, you'll probably get delayed again, possibly even longer than this time. Which means cycle six won't start until late summer, if not later."

That was longer than I thought. I knew another delay would be a possibility. I hoped that it wouldn't happen. Looks like my fears were founded in reality.

Dr. Jurgens continued, "You also have to ask yourself if you believe all the cancer was wiped out with the first four cycles. If not, you have to ask yourself if two more cycles will get the rest of it, knowing both will be a reduced dose of chemo."

"The first two cycles are more important than the last two," he went on, "You made it through four cycles."

We were silent for a few seconds, pondering our options.

"What would you do?" I asked him.

"If it were me, I'd stop after four cycles. The risks of continuing quickly start to outweigh the benefits. What we *do* know is that if you continue, it'll be at a half dose. You'll get delayed again at the end of the cycles, and your blood counts will drop to even lower levels, which carry other dangers in and of themselves."

"What we don't know," he went on, "is if there is any cancer left. There's no way to know. It's a gamble. In my opinion, you've got the odds in your favor. If it were *me*, I'd be fine with being done. But, that's up to you."

I looked at Kayleigh, motioning with my eyes for what she thought. "It's your decision, Babe," she told me, "But I agree with Dr. Jurgens. I don't want to risk it."

I looked back at Dr. Jurgens. "Okay then. Looks like I'll be done! I'd still like to get Dr. Lachance's opinion on the matter before we make this final, though."

"I'll email him when we're done here," Dr. Jurgens said. "But I'm sure he'll be okay with your decision as well. I'll have my nurse call you when he responds. Is there anything else?"

I sighed with relief. This ordeal was finally over – and much earlier than I was expecting. "No, I think we're good to go," I replied. I looked at my wife, "Babe? Anything from you?"

"No, I'm good too," she told both of us. Then she looked at Dr. Jurgens, "Thank you for everything."

"My pleasure," he replied. "Good luck to you both! Hopefully I never see you again." We all laughed as he shook our hands and left the room.

Kayleigh and I sat there for a few moments. We were both overjoyed. She squeezed my leg and pulled me in for a kiss.

"Yay!" she squealed, "You're done!"

"I know, right? What a ride!"

We got up and walked out of the exam room, hand-in-hand. We made our way out through the lobby and into the parking lot. It was surreal, like we were in a dream. Our nightmare was finally over. Now what? I had gotten used to this new version of my life. Moving on is going to be bittersweet.

Once in the car, I called my boss to share the news with him. He had asked me to call after our appointment to let him know how it went.

I shared with him our conversation with Dr. Jurgens, and that treatment was now over.

"That's great news!" he said, "congratulations!"

"Thanks," I replied. "I've been looking forward to this day for a long time."

"I bet," he replied. "I must say I wasn't expecting this. You kind of took me by surprise."

He paused for a moment before continuing, "So, I have your email pulled up here. I've been working with upper management to answer your thoughts and questions about the return to work plan we presented to you last week. I wasn't going to send it to you until you were done with treatment, but since you're now done, I'll send it."

"Fair warning, though," he continued, "you're not going to like parts of what it says."

He paused again, then went on, "I can send it now and we can talk through it, or I can send it after we hang up and we can talk in person once you've gathered your thoughts. Which would you prefer?"

"Send it later," I answered. I wasn't good with talking through heavy issues while emotional.

"Okay. Sounds good. Congrats again!"

By this time we had arrived at home and Kayleigh left me in the car to finish the conversation. I sat quietly, wondering what the email would say that I wasn't going to like.

I opened the door and headed into the house, checking my email on my phone to see if it had been sent yet. Kayleigh saw the look on my face.

"What's wrong?"

"He said I'm not going to like parts of what the email says. I'm nervous and scared."

"Go lie down on our bed. Take some time to decompress. I'm sure it'll be fine."

I went to our room, closed the door and laid on our bed. I checked my email every few minutes, waiting feverishly for it to come in.

I'm not sure how long I was in there, but Kayleigh came in and sat on the bed, rubbing my back. "Go play outside with the girls," she suggested. "It'll take your mind off of it. I'll make supper."

I nodded in agreement. I put my phone back in my pocket after I stood up. I started walking towards the bedroom door.

"Aren't you forgetting something?" Kayleigh asked sarcastically.

"Huh?"

"This," she gave me a big hug. I gladly hugged her back.

"It'll be fine, Honey! Stop worrying about it."

"I know. I'll try," I replied as I made my way outside to play with the girls.

Playing with them was a good distraction. We had fun running around and climbing on the playset. Eventually, Kayleigh called us in for dinner.

Towards the end of the meal, I pulled my phone out to check my email again. There it was. He finally sent it.

"Put your phone down!" Kayleigh scolded, "not at the dinner table."

I was breaking one of the cardinal rules of the house: no electronics at the dinner table.

"But the email just came in!" I pleaded.

"It can wait till we're done."

She was right. I sighed as I tucked my phone back in my pocket until we finished eating. As the girls were cleaning up, Kayleigh told me it was okay to read the email. I fumbled my phone back out and quickly pulled open the email.

What I read was devastating. My title was being changed to an entry level position. My new supervisor would be the Creative Director, the guy I helped hire back in 2010.

I was livid. My whole body was shaking. I gave the phone to Kayleigh so she could read the email. She was just as ticked.

They're demoting me? The guy with cancer. The guy who's entire life has been turned upside down. The guy who helped build this company from nothing. That's a dick-thing to do.

I couldn't think straight. All I saw was red. I was pissed. My job satisfaction dropped to zero in a heartbeat. I instantly hated the company. I hated my colleagues. I hated the leadership team. I hated everything.

"Go lay down," Kayleigh advised again. "Take some time to calm down. I'll clean up out here. I'm sure they had their reasons."

I slammed our bedroom door with a thunderous bang, and whipped my phone at the bed. I put my pillow over my face and screamed at the top of my lungs. I wanted to curl up and die.

After everything I've done for that company, this is how they repay me? With a demotion? Was this their plan all along?

I was still shaking. I screamed again into my pillow. Trying to calm myself down, I took a few deep breaths. My eyes were closed as I took several deep breaths through my nose. After a few minutes, I picked up my phone and read the email again. Then again. And again.

What have I done wrong? They're punishing me for getting cancer.

Then my logical brain stepped into my thoughts.

Nobody is punishing you. Kayleigh's right. I'm sure they have their reasons. The email said this is for mine and the company's best interest at this time. At this time. So it's not permanent, right?

I began to calm down. A little.

Nobody is that evil. Who would demote a guy with cancer?

I'm not sure how long I was in there. Kayleigh knocked on the door. Apparently it locked when I slammed it shut.

"Can I come in?"

"Sorry! Didn't realize the door had locked."

"You okay?" she asked as I opened the door.

"I don't know. I'm just pissed. I can't even think straight."

"I get it. I would feel the same way, too. Why don't you

come out and spend some time with us. It'll take your mind off of it for a while."

All I wanted to do was lie in my bed and mope, to wallow in my anger. Misery loves company, after all. But, logic won again. I begrudgingly left my phone in our room and went out to spend some time with my family.

We put a movie on until bedtime. Kayleigh had cleaned up the mess from supper, did the dishes and wiped the counters down. That was usually my job. I cleaned up the kitchen and did the dishes, she did the laundry. It was a nice little arrangement. We've had it ever since we moved in together. She doesn't like dishes, and I don't like laundry. It worked out well for us. I felt grateful. She did my job for me that night. I was in no mood to do it.

There was a constant pit in my stomach - even during the movie. After the girls were in bed, my mind wandered back to the email. I was so blinded with anger that I couldn't see the forest for the trees.

I read the email over and over again. Analyzing every word; every nuance. It only served as fuel for my anger.

I didn't sleep at all that night. I tossed and turned, my heart was pounding through my chest. I'm sure my pulse was well over a hundred. No matter what I did, I couldn't get my mind off that damn email.

In fact, I didn't sleep very well for the next few nights. Each night got progressively better, but my anger was so strong that it didn't allow me to calm down so I could think clearly and logically.

The next day, I called my father. I told him I wanted his advice about something going on at work. Dads are great like that, aren't they? I asked if we could come down to visit that night with the kids. Mom and Kayleigh would hang out with the "the grands" (as my parents call them) while Dad and I went out to chat.

He took me to dinner. I let him read the email, and the return to work plan. My dad has a knack for setting his emotions aside and thinking logically.

"Try putting yourself in their shoes," he told me. "Like Kayleigh said, they probably have a good reason for doing this. The email said it's for your best interest. Have some faith. You've been there for over a decade, and have been a great employee for them."

I sighed. "I know. You're right. It's just so hard to not assume the worst about it."

"Travis, that's normal!" Dad replied. "It's human nature to assume the worst. Don't beat yourself up over it. I don't like it either, but you need to give them the benefit of the doubt. A little trust will go a long way."

His words were salt in an open wound. Not because I didn't believe him, but because I knew he was right. It all boiled down to a lack of trust. I hadn't been at the office full-time for almost three months. My interactions with my colleagues were limited at best, and only through email. The last few weeks, I hadn't worked at all; I hadn't spoken to anyone at work.

As the next few days progressed, I slowly came to a realization. I figured out why this was happening. I stopped calling it a demotion. Instead, I called it a "Status Change." Once I started thinking of it in those terms, things became clear. They weren't reducing my salary. The only things that changed were my title and direct supervisor, and it really was in my best interest.

Before I stopped working, when chemo brain was in full effect, I wasn't doing the job of my old title, Director of Marketing Services. I wasn't directing anything or anybody. I wasn't innovating. I wasn't bringing change, implementing new ideas, or practices. I wasn't thinking of the big picture and how to move the company forward. All of those things are the core values of our company. Each employee is graded on them during their reviews.

I used to do all of those things, and then chemo brain kicked in and screwed it all up. Before I left, I was doing entry-level work because that's all I was cognitively capable of.

They wanted to bring me back in at the same level I left. Entry level. If they brought me back at the same level I was before I got cancer, they'd be setting me up to fail. Then, I'd either get a real demotion, or I'd face termination. The change in status really *was* in my best interest.

Once I came to that realization, I felt awful for jumping to conclusions and thinking the things I did. Many companies wouldn't have even held a job for me. They'd have left me with my long term disability and no job to come back to. Sorry, Kid. Good luck!

I'm grateful to Leighton Enterprises. Like I said in the beginning, working for a small, local company, is one of the best things that's ever happened to me. They've proven it to me time and time again over the last decade, and I'm sure they'll continue to prove it to me over the coming years.

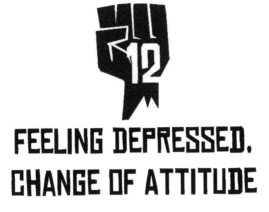

FEELING DEPRESSED.
CHANGE OF ATTITUDE

After I started working from home for a couple of weeks, my depression began to worsen. I was lonely. My colleagues' lives and jobs kept moving forward while my career was on pause. I would go in each week for leadership team meetings and Friday Beerstorming meetings, but it wasn't enough to just "be there." I wanted to be involved like I was before; doing work that makes a difference for our clients. Doing work I loved. When I stopped working entirely because of what chemotherapy did to my brain, my depression only got worse.

I really wanted to be involved in what was going on each day. I helped build that company from just two of us to more than sixteen over the last five years. I had a lot of blood, sweat and tears into that place; so to put everything on hold was the hardest thing I've ever had to do. More difficult than diagnosis, surgery, radiation and chemo combined. It was like being forced to sit on the sidelines and watch your baby grow up, powerless to teach, lead, or guide.

You'd think that surgery, radiation and chemo would be the worst parts of dealing with cancer. They're not. The emotional fallout from having everything I loved about my job taken away from me, having my life turned upside-down, and my family routine thrown out the window, is far worse. My body healed up just fine. My brain takes much longer to heal. My emotions take much longer to heal.

They say cancer is a yearlong battle of suck, and then life can return to normal, as it was before. They're wrong. It'll be at least two years for me by the time I'm fully back in the saddle and able to do the things I was capable of before I had cancer. My life will never be the same again. It's almost as if I now had two versions of my life: pre-cancer and post-cancer. Kind of like B.C. and A.D. They're two different eras of our civilization. I now have two different eras of my life, and I didn't like the post-cancer era.

Since I'm not there yet, I'm not sure if I'll ever be mentally capable of doing the job I left. That thought scares the hell out of me. To possibly be incapable of doing what I used to do is a demoralizing thought, especially since I don't know how long it'll take to get there, if ever.

I was afraid of missing out on what was going on at the office. Brené Brown, New York Times Best Selling Author, calls this F.O.M.O. – Fear of Missing Out.

She posted the following on her Facebook page:

The "fear of missing out" is what happens when scarcity slams into shame. FOMO lures us out of our integrity with whispers about what we could or should be doing. FOMO's favorite weapon is comparison. It kills gratitude and replaces it with "not enough." We answer FOMO's call by saying YES when we mean NO. We abandon our path and our boundaries and those precious adventures that hold meaning for us so we can prove that we aren't missing out.

But we are. We're missing out on our own lives. Every time we say YES because we're afraid of missing out, we say NO to something. That something may be a big dream or a short nap. We need both. Courage to stay our course and gratitude for our path will keep us grounded and guide us home.

-Brené Brown

I didn't realize how debilitating that would be until I went through it. I was so afraid of missing out on things going on at work. I feared missing out on being involved with the leadership team; what they were discussing, the decisions they were making to take our company to the next level. I feared missing out on client meetings, and being involved in projects. I had a fear of missing out of my colleagues' lives and being there every day. I was so engrained with my fear of missing out at work that I was missing out on the most important things going on right in front of my nose: my life, my kids, my wife. Recovering from brain cancer.

The fear of missing out only served to drive me deeper into depression. The more I tried to hang on to what I was missing out on, the more depressed I became.

Because of my time at home, I started assuming the worst about my colleagues, especially the leadership team. The people I was closest to were the ones I found myself despising. I hated how I felt that way towards them. They've been nothing but gracious to me during all of this, they didn't deserve to have me feel like this towards them. They never actually did or said anything to make my feelings justified.

I just interpreted what they told me in the most negative and awful ways possible. I'd take something that was said and twist it to what it could possibly mean and how it would affect me the worst. All of this was because I was so insecure about being home and not working.

I didn't feel like I was wanted or even missed. When I'd go in each week for our leadership team meetings, or Friday Beerstorming sessions, I felt like they'd talk as if I wasn't needed or even wanted. They didn't tell me I was missed or make me feel like I was needed around the office each day. They did when I first came back after surgery and radiation. For some twisted reason, I wanted them to keep telling me. I'm sure they would've if I had been transparent about what I was feeling and what I was going through, but I didn't. If I would have simply communicated, I could have avoided all of this.

Instead, I bottled up my emotions and let my negativity run wild in my head. I started assuming the worst about my co-workers and had no desire to change.

Brené Brown has her own version of this. She calls it

"creating your own story." She tells of a time when she did it with one of her employees. She was on the verge of firing this person, simply because she had created her own story in her own head without so much as talking to that person. Against all odds, she decided to have a face-to-face, heart-to-heart talk. Turns out, it was all a big misunderstanding. She was so ingrained in her own story, that she was willing to fire one of her employees over it.

That's what I was doing. I was writing my own story in my head about my colleagues and what they thought of me, and how they viewed me. I'd constantly find myself playing out scenarios in my head that would never actually happen. Don't you just love it when your brain does that to you? This only served as fuel for my anger, bitterness, and depression. It even got to a point where I seriously considered quitting.

Screw it all! I thought. *I'll be better off somewhere else where I'm actually cared about!*

It sounds silly, doesn't it? That's because it was silly. And stupid, and immature. I brought it all on myself, too.

On one of our trips down to Rochester for a follow-up MRI, I had a conversation with my wife that made me realize something: I had an attitude problem. It was a piss-poor attitude, in fact. The one who needed to change was me. Together, we made a list of three categories of things I can do each week to change my attitude and fix my depression:

1. Things I can do to better myself.
2. Household projects to keep me busy.
3. Ways to show sincere appreciation to those around me.

I put a handful of things in each category. I committed to doing at least one thing from each category each week. This would keep me busy, keep my mind active and my thoughts positive. The only person I could change was myself, but I had to *want* to change before I could *start* to change.

I had myself convinced that, since I had cancer and was going through chemotherapy, everyone should feel sorry for me. They should make me feel missed, make me feel needed and wanted. They should try to make me happy.

I didn't consciously think those things. They grew in my subconscious until they became reality through my attitude and thoughts. As the saying goes, "Your thoughts become your attitude, your attitude becomes your words, your words become your reputation and your reputation becomes your destiny."

I needed to change my attitude in order to cure my depression.

I don't mean to imply that people with mental illnesses like depression, bi-polar, obsessive compulsive disorder, etc. can simply change their attitude and be all better. It's not like there is a magical Attitude Change Pill that will cure those diseases. Those folks have a chemical imbalance in their brain which requires medication to fix. An attitude adjustment won't fix it for them. Thinking about things positively and trying to have a good attitude certainly will help, but it won't cure the disorder.

In my case, I got depressed from sitting at home all day with nothing but my negative thoughts to bring me down. I believe there are two ways to get depressed: situational and clinical. I had situational depression. The things I mentioned above are clinical disorders. They're very different things and are treated very differently.

I've been situationally depressed twice in my life. The first time I was in my late teens.

I was just fired from my first job as a cook for a local restaurant. Apparently, I was asking for too much time off in the summer. I gave my boss a four-month notice of the time I wanted to take off in the summer. Instead of saying no, or working with me on it, he fired me. Who does that?

I was just a kid and wanted to enjoy my summers. I wanted to take a week off to go on a church road trip. I wanted another two weeks off so I could volunteer at a summer camp. I wanted a long weekend to go to a music festival. All in all, I was asking for about a month's worth of time off in the summer, and I had given four months' advance notice. I wasn't a full-time employee either. All my boss had to do was say no, and I would have come in to work.

He didn't even have the guts to tell me to my face. He used the passive-aggressive angle and just took me off the schedule. Was I just supposed to get the hint that I didn't work there anymore? C'mon, man. Grow a pair.

I actually had to come in to the restaurant and ask him why I wasn't scheduled anymore. I told him I didn't need all that time off. I was willing to pare it down to the music festival and the road trip. He wasn't willing to negotiate.

I filed for unemployment. My boss contested it. I won.

That was also the same summer when Kayleigh and I had an unplanned pregnancy; our first daughter, Alexis.

During this time, I was volunteering at a Christian radio station every Saturday night for a Christian rock radio show. I had been doing it since I was 15. I was the Executive Producer of the show – I was basically the guy in charge of everything, which isn't saying much because the staff were all volunteers.

The radio station stayed out of our show. They lets us pick the music, arrange prizes and contests, and even put on concerts. Looking back, I'm surprised they gave a group of teenagers so much leeway. Knowing what I know now about radio, I wouldn't have done that.

Kayleigh was one of the volunteers. We couldn't hide the pregnancy any longer because she was starting to show. We emailed the staff and let them know she was pregnant.

Lo and behold, the new Program Director who started just a few months prior, who had nothing to do with our show, sat us down and fired me. I was on the payroll outside of the volunteer hours on Saturday night. I ran the board back in the studio for college football games, which they paid me for.

He told Kayleigh she was welcome to stay. She didn't, obviously. Why would she?

This was the same guy who knocked up his wife before they were married. Talk about being a hypocrite.

So, there I was. Jobless with a baby on the way, and not mature enough to know what to do. I had no idea how to raise a baby. Nothing in my life was seeming to go my way.

Kayleigh was in her senior year of high school. I was in

my first year of college. My plans for life were just thrown out the window. I got depressed. I also learned that you can't plan your own life. You can make a rough outline - a general direction – but that's about as good as it'll get. It never fails that a wrench will get thrown into your plan and you'll have to manage around it. Sometimes, that wrench will change your plan entirely. An unplanned pregnancy did that for us.

But, time heals all wounds. I found another restaurant job a couple months later. We talked to our parents about the pregnancy. We made it work, and we both finished college. The whole thing turned into one of the biggest blessings of our lives. Without it, we wouldn't have our oldest daughter.

Fast forward to 2005. I was hired at Leighton Broadcasting, so I quit my job at the restaurant. Kayleigh and I were married in 2006 and our life has been great ever since. Not to say our relationship has been ladybugs and roses the whole time. We've had our issues like every married couple has, but we worked them out because we made a promise to be together till death do us part. We both took that vow seriously. I can honestly say the last ten years of my life have been among the best.

Then, we found out I had brain cancer. That alone is enough to derail a relationship. When I started working from home, that's when my second bout with situational depression set in. Though, the seeds of it were sewn months before, likely during my time in Rochester for radiation.

Being in the Box

I've noticed over the years that given multiple possible interpretations of what someone says to you, we tend to assume the negative first. We judge ourselves by our intentions, and we judge others by their words and actions. When it comes to ourselves, we never assume the negative. We always have the best, most pure intentions in anything we do. Yet, we assume others have the worst possible intentions.

Think of it this way. Imagine you're stuck in rush hour traffic. Out of nowhere, the car in front of you cuts over two lanes of traffic to take the exit ramp, and you lay on the horn in self-righteous anger. What's your first thought?

Learn to drive, Moron! Pay attention to the road!

You instantly assume the worst. That driver is a moron who doesn't know how to drive.

How many other possibilities are there about that situation on the freeway? Dozens. Yet you jumped right to the worst one and assumed the negative about the other driver.

Isn't it possible that he just got word his wife was going into labor and had to veer off to get to the hospital in time? Sure it is.

Isn't it also possible that he or she simply wasn't paying attention? We're all guilty of drifting off to la-la land while driving. So why is that driver suddenly a moron when you've done the same thing many times before?

What if their kid threw up in the car? What if they forgot something and needed to turn around? What if, what if, what if.

There are dozens of possible reasons for that driver to

cut you off and take the first exit. But, you chose the worst reason. Why is that?

I think this is part of human nature; to always look out for number one. If you're not with me, you're against me. It's my way or the highway. We approach situations with a win or lose mindset. We need to win and the other person needs to lose. There are no other options.

This is actually a result of how we've evolved as humans. When we're afraid, nervous, or anxious, we're on high alert. For our ancestors, being on high alert was literally a matter of life or death.

Back when our people were simple-minded hunters and gatherers, they'd be sitting around a campfire in the dense forest. If they heard a twig snap in the darkness, they'd instantly spring into fight or flight mode. The men were on the ready with spears and rocks. The women were huddled around the fire, protecting the babies and children. All eyes on the lookout for danger. They *had* to assume the worst. It could be a lion or a bear, or a pack of hungry wolves circling the camp. Their lives depended on assuming the worst of the unknown.

This evolutionary trait helped us survive and evolve into our modern, technologically advanced society. It still serves us some use today.

Have you ever been lying in bed at night and hear a noise in the dark reaches of your home? We all have. You jump into an alert status. You're wide awake in a heartbeat. If you have kids, your first thought is about them, and what you would do if it came down to fisticuffs with an intruder. Your eyes are wide, ears alert. You're listening intently for more clues as to what the sound could be.

Most of the time, it's just the house settling, or a cat knocking something over haphazardly. That's what it typically is in our house: one of the damn cats getting into something. But still, we heard it and perked up. Our fight or flight instincts kicked in.

What if it was a burglar? Or what if it started a fire? What if someone broke in to kidnap one of our daughters? That's why we have a hockey stick next to our bed - to defend our family if it ever came down to it.

In other ways, that trait evolved causes us to always assume the worst of the unknown, which isn't so helpful these days.

I read a book a few years ago called *Leadership and Self-Deception* by The Arbinger Institute. It changed my life. I'm not kidding, either. It's written like a novel about a new manager recently hired at a company. It outlines a principle called "Being in the Box." What that boils down to, for me at least, is that other people can sense how you're *being* towards them. It also backed up my theory that people tend to assume the negative first. Yet, when it comes to yourself and your own intentions, you never start with the negative.

The book gives an example of a husband and wife lying in bed at night. Then, the baby starts crying from across the house. Both remain motionless, secretly hoping the other will get up.

I've had a long day at the office, the husband thinks to himself. *She should get up with the baby. Plus, I got up with the baby last night. It's her turn.*

Does he not know how my day has been? The wife ponders to herself. *I've been with the baby all day. He can get up this time.*

She's not moving. Doesn't she care that her child is screaming?

He's not moving. Doesn't he care that his child is screaming?

They both get up in a huff, angry at the other. Each is determined the other is in the wrong.

"Don't worry," the wife says sarcastically, "I'll get the baby...again!"

Then they begin to fight and bicker about who works harder, who cares more, who is more deserving of a break. Yet, neither had said *anything* up until that point. They just laid in bed and thought the worst about the other. They were creating their own stories in their minds. They were assuming the worst about each other.

That's the essence of being in the box towards somebody or towards a group of people. Once I realized I was "in the box" toward my colleagues, I could take steps to get myself out of that box.

What if they were in the box towards me? They might have been. I honestly don't know. But I can't control them or their behavior. I can only control me. Many of us at the office have read the book, and are familiar with the concept of being in the box towards someone. We knew what it meant and how to get out of the box. Like the book says, we can't control what other people think, say, or do. We can only control ourselves. Even if they were in the box towards me, there's nothing I could do about it.

Since I was thinking that my colleagues were not missing me, not making me feel wanted or needed, I acted in a manner to further those thoughts. When we have pre-determined blueprints about others in our head, we tend to act in a way to make them complete that blueprint. It's a self-fulfilling prophecy. I had a blueprint for each colleague and how I *thought* they viewed me. So, I acted accordingly around them, subconsciously trying to force their words and actions into my mental blueprint.

For me, every twig snap in the darkness was a pack of wolves prowling around my little fire, eager to devour me. Everyone was out to get me, and I was going to fight to the death to survive.

What did that actually look like in action? When I'd go in for meetings, I'd sit quietly and not say much. I'd give answers that were short and abrupt, almost rude. I'd complain to my boss about how "I'm really sensitive right now, so you need to be careful what you say around me because I take things very differently than I did before."

I refused to take control of my own circumstance. I was blaming everyone around me for not caring as much as I thought they should. I don't mean to imply that nobody cared. They just didn't care in ways I *wanted* them to. I was being selfish and arrogant. I felt like I deserved to feel that way. I had cancer after all. Those thoughts and feelings only served to drive me deeper into depression, and make me more and more angry, and more and more bitter.

No. What really needed to happen was that I had to change my attitude. Just because I have cancer, doesn't mean the world has to stop and lick *my* wounds. It's *my* job to get better. It's *my* job to change my attitude. It's *my* job to focus on me first. Never has that been more apparent than going through the final stages of chemotherapy and subsequent recovery.

So, I took steps to get out of the box. Once I started to

change my attitude, everyone else seemed to change, too. And, that's the thing: nobody else changed. The simple act of changing my attitude changed my entire worldview and how I saw and interpreted others' words and actions. It was as if I was looking at the world through a whole new lens. A happy, joyful lens instead of a depressed lens. Pretty cool, huh?

Remember when I told you about that book I kept putting off reading? It was *The 7 Habits of Highly Effective People* by Stephen R. Covey. I started reading it during this period of my life. This is why I kept putting it off. I was *meant* to read it at this point in my cancer journey.

I'm not someone who believes that everything happens for a reason. I don't believe that God, or some other omniscient being, *allowed* me to get brain cancer just to teach me something. It's like when you're late for work, and someone says to you, "You were late for a reason. Maybe God was saving you from a terrible car accident. You should be thankful!"

That's baloney. What about all those other people who *did* get into car accidents that morning? Did they just not pray hard enough? Did they not believe enough? Did God just love you more than he loves them? No. Shit just happens. That's life.

On the other hand, though, sometimes things happen that we can't quite explain. Like why I kept putting off reading that book for so long. I don't know why, but *something* kept telling me to put it off.

When I finally started reading it, the book changed my life. I've said that about a lot of books, and I've meant it about those books too. That's the power of a good book. It can change your life if you let it.

Because of that book, I was inspired to write a personal mission statement. Stephen Covey suggests that everyone should write their own, based on the values they hold most dear. Everyone's will be unique.

Here's mine:

- Put God and family are above all else.
- Never assume the negative about another.
- Be positive and joyful in all things.
- Do my best and forget the rest.
- Be financially independent; don't worry about money.
- Focus on things I can control.
- Never have a Fear of Missing Out.

Notice there's nothing in there about my job. I can't control what happens to that part of my life. It's for that reason I chose to leave it out of my mission statement. Do I love my job? Yes. Can I control what happens to my career in the coming years? No.

I can only do my best - part of my mission statement - and hope it pays off in the long run. If not, I'll forget it and move on. I know, much easier said than done, especially when I care so deeply about my job, the company, and my colleagues.

I refer to this mission statement every day. Several times a day if I need to. I have it on my phone so it's always in my pocket for easy access. The mission statement is what I look at when I need to check my attitude, thoughts, or behavior. Whenever I need to check myself before I wreck myself, the mission statement is always there to slap me in the face.

"Get your shit together, Travis!" it screams. "You're better than this! Don't let your thoughts and attitude control you! You can do this!"

It's a work in progress, just like my life. My mission statement is never complete, and it's never incomplete. It's perfect for the current time in my life. I've made several revisions to it. I'll make more as I get older and my life priorities change.

Also in that book, Covey describes something called the stimulus/response phenomenon. It is based on Pavlov's findings in his experimentation with dogs. Ring a bell?

Sorry, I couldn't resist.

Covey explains that one of the biggest things separating us from animals is our ability to be self-aware. To think about thinking. Simply put, between the stimulus and the response, we have the freedom of choice. Animals do not. If you train a dog to expect food whenever a bell rings, it will always expect food when a bell rings. It has no choice in the matter. You could train it to respond to something else, but the dog is incapable of changing its response on its own accord.

Humans have the unique ability to interrupt the stimulus/response sequence and *choose* our response. For me, the stimulus was being home by myself, away from the job and people I so dearly loved. After a while, the response to that stimulus became negative thoughts, a piss-poor attitude, and ultimately, depression.

On that fateful trip down to Rochester with my wife, I had the realization that I – and only I – can *choose* how to respond to that stimulus. I chose to change my attitude. I was subconsciously blaming my circumstance - which was beyond my control - and letting it dictate my thoughts and attitudes. When I realized that I was the one the in driver's seat of the response, everything changed for the better.

Kayleigh has been a great sounding board for me to share my feelings. She isn't afraid to tell me how it is. She won't join my pity party just because she's my wife. In fact, she got angry with me on several occasions for not letting go of all the hurt, bitterness, and frustration.

Here's the final reason I was meant to read that book when I did: the author talks about the different kinds of centers people can have. Most people have one or two main centers. They might be Family-Centered, Spouse-Centered, Work-Centered, Possession-Centered, Pleasure-Centered, Friend/Enemy-Centered, Church-Centered, Self-Centered, or Money-Centered.

They get their sense of value and self-worth from their particular center. When I read the list, I didn't think I fit into any of those.

I place my values on non-worldly things. I'm not like those people he talks about, I thought to myself.

Each center has their benefits, but one huge drawback: nothing in life is permanent. If any of the things you place your center in go away, you lose. And nobody likes losing. You've built your house in sand. When the storms of life come and wash the sand away, you've got nothing left. No solid ground to stand on, no universal truths to live by. You start sinking in your own self-doubt. You question your value and worth. You question everything you've ever known to be true because everything you thought was true has turned out to be a lie.

It wasn't until I read the description of each type of center that I had a sickening realization: I am very much a Work-Centered person. Most of my self-worth and value came from my status at work, and being successful in my career. My title, my responsibilities, and the respect of others meant the world to me. I loved getting awards and accolades, and being praised for my work. I enjoyed being viewed as a thought leader and respected by my industry peers as "the guy with the answers."

It felt good to be recognized, promoted, and given awards for the work I took great pride in. I wanted to do a good job, to be successful. It made me feel good, and it boosted my self-esteem.

But, my idea of "success" was rooted in fallacy: in order to succeed, you need to climb the corporate ladder. Earn a bigger title, earn more money, and earn more responsibilities. Once you do those things, *then* you're successful. Because I believed that fallacy to be true, I had been trying to climb the corporate ladder ever since my career began.

It's not like I was a bully or anything. I treated those around me with respect, and didn't try to lie or cheat my way to the top. I worked hard and earned it the honest way. My parents taught me the value of hard work, and I took that teaching very seriously. If someone around me was promoted, I was sincerely happy for them. I knew that if I worked hard, and was a loyal employee, it would pay off in the long run. And it did.

I'm not saying you shouldn't work hard and enjoy what you do. There's nothing wrong with that. There's nothing wrong with wanting to earn more money and to be more successful in your career and hone your craft. Just don't put your self-worth in those things. They won't last. I know first-hand.

It's not like I wanted to have success over everyone else, or that I wanted to be better than my colleagues. That's not it at all. I actually took great joy in seeing those around me succeed. I enjoyed teaching and mentoring them to do so, and I enjoyed learning new things from them. Anyone can be a teacher, regardless of their position in the company. I *wanted* those around me to be better than me. As the saying goes, "hire people who are better than you."

For me, my self-esteem lived and died with my job. It was all inward. When I had my title, responsibilities, and respect taken away, my life fell apart. That's why I got depressed. It had very little to do with my cancer. Cancer was just the catalyst.

Since then, I've worked hard to make my life have a different center. A "Principle-Center," as Stephen Covey calls it. To really get my self-worth from things in life that matter and won't go away. That's why I created my personal mission statement. Those are the items I want to find value in, to get my self-esteem from. God and family. Hard work. Choosing joy. Being financially secure.

Everyone will have different things that matter to them. For me, those are what matter. They're universal truths for those who want to live a happy life. I was placing my value in the wrong place. And when it all came crashing down, so did I.

To this day, it's still a work in progress. It always will be. I still slip up sometimes. It happens more often than sometimes. It happens rather frequently, actually. I've got brain cancer, after all. It's easy to fall back into being down in the dumps about my situation. When I slip up though, I can check myself. Check my thoughts. Check my attitude. Interrupt the stimulus and response with a choice to be happy and thankful. To *choose* joy over sorrow.

It's the most difficult thing I've ever done. But, anything worth doing won't be easy. So, I'm choosing the difficult path – the path that leads to happiness and fulfillment – not the path leading to despair, and depression. I refuse to wallow away in self-pity.

My chosen path is littered with rocks and obstacles. What else will I encounter on my journey? I can't imagine anything any worse than brain cancer – but, who knows. The death of my wife, or one of my girls would probably top it, but at least I'm better prepared now for whatever life throws my way.

I didn't let my depression get the best of me. I didn't let my lack of joy take me out for good. I have a beautiful family. My parents, siblings, and in-laws are the best a guy could ask for. I adore my girls. My bride is the love of my life. If I can focus on those things, then I'll be fine no matter what happens. It certainly won't be easy, but nobody ever said it would be easy.

It will be worth it, though. Well worth it.

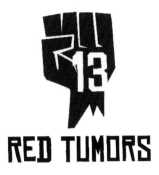

RED TUMORS

Even after all this time, it still sounds weird saying I have brain cancer. I was only 30-years old when I was diagnosed. The nice thing about brain cancer is that it cannot spread to other parts of the body. That's also the bad thing about brain cancer, it can't spread! It's a double edged sword.

Honestly though, I'm not sure I'd rather have any other type of cancer, because knowing what I know now, I can't say that lung cancer would be better. How about pancreatic cancer, or prostate cancer? They're all bad, but brain cancer is a walk in the park so far. At least it was looking back at my journey. Overall, I didn't get *that* sick from chemo or radiation. I was never on my death bed or anything close to it. All things considered, chemo brain aside, this has been pretty easy in retrospect.

Sure, it was by far the worst thing I've ever had to deal with, but I survived and I'm stronger because of it.

A lot went through my mind when we found out the tumor was a Grade III Glioma. Grade IV is the worst. The grading scale is I-IV. Grade I is only found in children. Grade II is what we were hoping for. With Grade II, while technically it's still cancerous, it grows so slowly that they just watch it over the next several years before deciding upon a treatment plan.

It was the night before our appointment with our neurologist, Dr. Lachance, when we read the pathology report. The Mayo Clinic has a neat app my wife and I installed on our phones. You can login and view your entire patient history. That's where we found the pathology report.

It was a Grade III Oligoastrocytoma. You could've heard the sound of my broken heart as it shattered into a million little pieces.

I didn't sleep that night, tossing and turning. I cried my eyes dry. I got up and went to the bathroom three or four times. My mind was a rollercoaster of thoughts, mostly negative. I couldn't help my brain from going there, despite my desperate pleas to make it stop. My heart was banging out of my chest. No matter how I laid, my ear drums pounded with nervousness. I saw every hour on the clock tick by in slow motion.

What is he going to say tomorrow? Do I have three to four years to live? Seven to nine? Surely a Grade III Glioma can't be that good. I'm going to die. What about my kids? Harper won't even remember her Daddy! Alexis won't get to have me walk her down the aisle. Tatum is so confused about what's going on, will she even remember me? Kayleigh, my wife! What will she do without me? Will she remarry? How long till she does? I love her so much. I don't want to be selfish, but I don't want her to get married to someone else either.

I wish I had never read that damn pathology report. They don't put anything in there about prognosis.

It was 7 a.m. when we got up. Longest. Night. Ever. It didn't help that our appointment wasn't until 3:15 that afternoon. We found ways to kill time. We watched television in our room until we had to check out. Then we meandered around downtown Rochester, where the Mayo Clinic is located. We visited some shops, perused Barnes & Noble, and then stopped at Starbucks for some coffee.

Both of us were dragging from the sleepless night before. I had a headache from the surgery a few days prior. I could barely think straight. Being dead tired on top of that made both things worse. We sat quietly in the coffee shop. Kayleigh was reading a book. I closed my eyes and tried to get some much needed rest, while my coffee got cold next to me.

It was finally 3:00. We headed up to the 8th Floor of the Gonda Building to check-in for my appointment with Dr. Lachance. We found out that was delayed because he had to be at the hospital for something urgent. We waited in the lobby for nearly two hours.

It was the day Robin Williams died. The internet and social media were buzzing with the news. I remember it like it was yesterday. Not because of Robin Williams, but because this meeting could change my life forever.

I couldn't sit still. My legs and fingers were fidgety. My heart raced. I got up and used the restroom several times. I'm not sure where the liquid kept coming from. I paced back and forth in the waiting area.

After an eternity, we were finally called back.

Dr. Lachance asked about my surgery and was impressed with how quickly I recovered.

He did the same neurological exam that we did back in July. I didn't fare so well this time. My right side was noticeably more sluggish. I couldn't tap my right foot as quickly as I could the left. I couldn't hold my right arm straight out in front of me without it beginning to tremble. My facial expressions were still flat. These would all get much better in the coming weeks and months, but it was obvious I had just had my brain cut open.

He also asked me to read a passage from a magazine, and then tell him what the whole article was about. He was testing my cognitive ability to extrapolate a larger meaning from a small chunk of information.

I read the words on the page, out loud to him, but none of them had any meaning to me. They were just empty words on a page. I struggled. I had to pause on several words before reading them.

"What do you think the story is about?" he asked.

I sat quiet for a few moments, struggling to piece together something that would have been so easy a few days ago.

"I don't know. Canoeing? Camping?" I saw those words in the snippet he had me read. I hoped I was right.

"Not quite." He replied, flipping to the first page of the article. "It's about Northern Minnesota. Those are things you can do in Northern Minnesota, but they're not what the article is actually about."

He then got started on what the pathology report said – something we saw the night before already, so it wasn't anything new for us.

It was 5:30 when we left our appointment.

My prognosis is 15 years - based on a study done 15 years ago. In it, about 75% of the participants with the same type of tumor as me have shown no signs of regrowth over that time frame. So really, I don't have a prognosis. I could live to be 105 years old. Or, I could step off the curb tomorrow and get hit by a bus.

I have a love/hate relationship with the practice of giving a patient their prognosis. On one hand, it gives them something solid to rely on. There's a level of relief in knowing what your outlook is. In a morbid sense, there's some comfort in knowing how long you might live.

On the other hand, it's just a number based on a study and median survival rates when specific criteria are met. I'm sure there's some formula they run for each patient and it spits back a possible prognosis for that individual based on their specific condition.

The Mayo Clinic published a study on June 22nd, 2015 in the New England Journal of Medicine. It was titled, "Glioma Groups Based on 1p/19q, IDH, and TERT Promoter Mutations in Tumors." I know, typical name for a fancy medical journal publication.

I was one of the 1,087 gliomas that contributed data to the study. They broke down various grade II and III gliomas based on the genetic makeup of the tumor. Each was given a color code: Blue, Green, Pink, Red, Yellow, and Purple. I was a Red Tumor.

Each color represented a specific combination of genetic mutations: 1p/19q Codeletion, IDH Mutated, and/or TERT Promoted. The presence or absence of any of these determined the color group. I was a "triple positive" with IDH Mutation, 1p/19q codeletion, and TERT Promoted. I'm no genetics whiz, so I'm not sure what each of those actually mean, but I have learned quite about tumor genetics over the last year.

So, what does a red tumor mean? I'm glad you asked.

A red tumor has the greatest long-term outlook before signs of regrowth appeared.

The study has 10 years' worth of data. Dr. Lachance showed us the graph, and the red tumor group had a 75% survival rate at the 10-year mark.

"What happens after that?" I asked.

"Well, we have studies from 15 years ago that show the same trend," Dr. Lachance replied. "The line continues to level off."

"What's up with the green group?" I asked, pointing to the graph. The green line took a nose dive down to the 5% range right at the 3-year mark.

"We're glad you're not a Green Tumor," he smiled. "Those folks didn't fare very well long-term. But, you'll be here for a long time!"

Tumors with only TERT promotion were the worst for long term survival. They're the Green Tumors. Telomerase reverse transcriptase (TERT) is part of an enzyme in our DNA.

When our cells divide, they breakdown in the process. This is one of the reasons we age, because our cells breakdown the more and more they divide. TERT enzymes bind to our cells and prevent them from breaking down, thus making those cells fundamentally immortal. When TERT enzymes are present in cancer, the tumor is essentially indestructible. Chemotherapy and radiation have very little effect on TERT-only tumors, which is why the lifespan of those patients is rarely more than three years.

Those tumors with only the IDH mutation and 1p/19q codeletion had a medium survival rate. When you add in the TERT promotion with the other mutations, it works wonders for long term survival. It doesn't make any sense to me either. Why would an indestructible tumor suddenly become very susceptible to radiation and chemo? I didn't ask, but I didn't really care. I'm just grateful I was in the red group.

My wife and I were both overjoyed after hearing this.

Honestly, I'm not that worried about it because it's outside of my control. Remember my personal mission statement? One of the items is to focus on things I can control. So, that's what I'm choosing to do. If I could control what would happen to me over the next fifteen years, I'd certainly not choose this.

Never before have I come face-to-face with my own mortality. It's like holding a poker hand and seeing your own death in the cards. There's nothing you can do but to play it out. Knowing what I know, would I still play my hand differently?

I'm not sure, honestly. I was simply dealt a shitty hand, and I'm doing my best (another part of my mission statement) to play it out.

Just imagine how far medicine will be in fifteen years. How about just two years from now, or five, or ten? Maybe there'll be a cure, or more effective treatment options than radiation and chemotherapy. The strides we're making in understanding how cancer works are mind-blowing.

I've learned to not take life too seriously. You'll never make it out alive, anyways. It's just not worth it to get worked up over something completely out of your control. I learned that the hard way. I'm sure I'll do it again. Then I'll refer to my personal mission statement, and it'll kick my ass back into the right mindset like it always does.

I've had some great things happen to me, and some really awful things happen to me. Brain cancer is on the top of the list of awful things. If you focus on the great parts in life – the parts that truly matter in the grand scheme of things, the awful parts won't seem so bad.

There are so many great things in this world more deserving of our time and attention. Things like family, and friends. Hard work. Doing your best at everything, and not being afraid to fail. Keeping your promises and being honest all the time. Those are the things that really matter in life.

Did brain cancer derail my life? Yes. Did it take me off course for good? Hell no. I won't let it. I can't control it, but I *can* control how I respond to it. That, right there, is the biggest lesson I've learned through all of this. We are in control of how we respond to things. To anything. Even life debilitating things like brain cancer.

I believe the sun also rises.
Dries our tears, bringing the blue skies of day.
I believe the sun also rises.
Lighting our past, driving the darkness away.
So far away, so far away.
  -Brave Saint Saturn

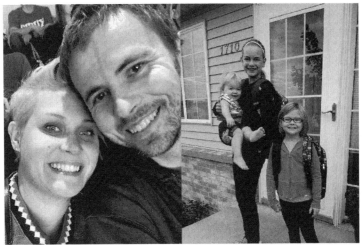

On the left, my wife and I at a Sioux Hockey Game in Grand Forks. On the right, my three gorgeous daughters on the first day of school in 2015.

I've been done with treatment for several months, but my life will never be the same again. I have follow-up MRI scans every six months at the Mayo Clinic for the foreseeable future. Eventually, we'll change to yearly scans for the rest of my life.

Every time we go down for a scan, we have to prepare for the worst and hope for the best. We didn't choose this life, but we can choose how to deal with it.

With my wife and kids by my side, I can take on anything life throws my way.

Thanks for reading.

Please follow me on Twitter: @stompwampa

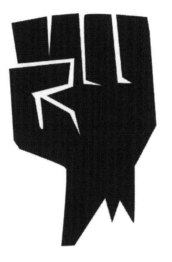

Made in the USA
Lexington, KY
09 February 2016